The Compleat Surgeon

by Charles Gabriel Le Clerc

THE

PREFACE.

So great a number of Treatises of Surgery, as well Ancient as Modern, have been already publish'd, that a plenary Satisfaction seems to have been long since given on this Subject, even to the Judgment of the most curious Inquirers: But if it be consider'd that a young Surgeon ought always to have in view the first Principles of this Noble Art explain'd after a familiar and intelligible manner, it will be soon acknowledg'd that there is good reason to set about the Work anew: For besides that the Writings of the Ancients being so voluminous, are not portable, they are also very intricate and confus'd; nay the whole Art has been so far improv'd and brought to perfection by able Masters in the present Age, that they are now almost become unprofitable.

Some Modern authors have set forth certain small Tracts, which only explain a few Chirurgical Operations, and on that account deserve only the Name of Fragments. Indeed the Works of some others seem to be sufficiently compleat, but are printed in so large Volumes, and contain so many Discourses altogether foreign from the principal Subject, that they have almost the same Inconveniences with those of the Ancients. Therefore the Reader is here presented with a small Treatise of Surgery, yet very plain and perspicuous, in a portable Volume; being free from a Multiplicity of impertinent Words, and containing every thing of moment that has been producd by the most approv'd Authors both Ancient and Modern.

An Introduction is made into the Matter by small Colloquies or Dialogues, to the end that the young Student may be at first lead as it were by the Hand; but as soon as he has attain'd to a considerable Progress in these Studies, this innocent and puerile manner of speaking is abandon'd, to conduct him in good earnest to the most sublime Heights of so admirable an Art; to which purpose, after having penetrated into its first Rudiments and Grounds, he is well instructed in Anatomy, and furnish'd with a general Idea of Wounds and Tumours, which are afterward treated of in particular: He is also taught a good Method of curing Wounds made by Gun-shot, the Scurvy, and all sorts of Venereal Diseases: From thence he is introduced into the Practice of all manner of Chirurgical Operations in Fractures and Luxations; together with the use of their respective Dressings and Bandages.

At the end of the Work is added a compleat Chirurgical Dispensatory, shewing the Method of preparing such Medicinal Compositions as are chiefly us'd in the Art of Surgery; so that upon the whole Matter, it may be justly affirm'd, that this little Manual has all the Advantages of the Ancient and Modern Writings on the same Subject, and is altogether free from their Superfluities and Defects.

* * * * *

{1}

THE

Compleat Surgeon:

OR, THE

Whole ART

OF

SURGERY

Explain'd, &c.

* * * * *

CHAP. I.

Of the Qualifications of a Surgeon, and of the Art of Surgery.

Who is a Surgeon?

A Person skill'd in curing Diseases incident to Humane Bodies by a methodical Application of the Hand.

What are the Qualifications of a good Surgeon in general?

They are three in Number: viz. Skill in the Theory, Experience in the Practical part, and a gentle Application of the Hand.

Why ought a Surgeon to be skilful?

Because without a discerning Faculty he can have no certainty in what he doth.

Why must he be experienc'd?

Because Knowledge alone doth not endue him with a dexterity of Hand requisite in such a Person, which cannot be acquir'd but by Experience, and repeated Manual Operations.

Why must he be tender-handed?

To the End that by fit Applications he may asswage those Pains which he is oblig'd to cause his Patients to endure.

What is Chirurgery or Surgery?

It is an Art which shews how to cure the Diseases of Humane Bodies by a methodical Manual Application. The Term being derived from the Greek Word [Greek: Cheir], signifying a Hand and [Greek: Ergon], a Work or Operation.

After how many manners are Chirurgical Operations usually perform'd?

Four several ways.

Which be they?

I. Synthesis, whereby the divided Parts are re-united; as in Wounds. II. Diesis, that divides and separates those Parts, which, by their Union, hinder the Cure of Diseases, such is the continuity of Abscesses or Impostumes which must be open'd to let out the purulent Matter. III. Exesis, which draws out of the Body whatsoever is noxious or hurtful, as Bullets, Arrows, &c. IV. Prosthesis adds some Instrument or Body to supply {3} the defect of those that are wanting; such are Artificial Legs and Arms, when the Natural ones are lost. It also furnishes us with certain Instruments to help and strengthen weak Parts, such as Pessaries, which retain the Matrix in its proper place when it is fallen, Crutches to assist feeble Persons in going, &c.

What ought to be chiefly observed before the undertaking an Operation?

Four things; viz. 1. What the Operation to be perform'd is? 2. Why it is perform'd? 3. Whether it be necessary or possible? And 4. The manner of performing it.

How may we discern these?

The Operation to be perform'd may be known by its Definition; that is to say, by explaining what it is in it self: We may discover whether it ought to be done, by examining whether the Distemper cannot be cur'd otherwise: We may also judge whether it be possible or necessary, by a competent Knowledge of the Nature of the Disease, the Strength of the Patient, and the Part affected: Lastly, the manner of performing it may be found out, by being well vers'd in the Practice of Surgery.

What are the Fundamental Principles of Surgery?

They are Three in number: viz. 1. The knowledge of Man's Body. 2. That of the Diseases which require a Manual Operation. 3. That of proper Remedies and Helps upon every Occasion.

How may one attain to the Knowledge of Humane Bodies? {4}

By the study of Anatomy.

How may one learn to know the Distempers relating to Surgery, and the Remedies appropriated for them?

Two several ways; viz. 1. By the reading of good Books, and Instructions receiv'd from able Masters of that Art. 2. By practice and the Observation of what is perform'd by others upon the Bodies of their Patients.

What are the Diseases in general that belong to Surgery?

They are Tumours, Impostumes, Wounds, Ulcers, Fractures, Dislocations, and generally all sorts of Distempers whereto Manual Operations may be applyed.

What are the Instruments in general which are commonly used in Surgery for the curing of Diseases?

They are Five; viz. the Hand, Bandages, Medicines, the Incision-Knife, and Fire.

What is the general Practice which ought to be observ'd in the Application of these different helps?

Hippocrates teacheth us, in saying, that when Medicines are not sufficient, recourse may be had to the Incision-Knife, and afterward to Fire; intimating that we must proceed by degrees.

Are there any Distempers that may be cured by the Surgeon's Hand alone?

Yes, as when a simple and small Dislocation is only to be reduced.

* * * * *

{5}

CHAP. II.

Of Chirurgical Instruments, portable and not portable.

What do you call portable and not portable Instruments?

Portable Instruments are those which the Surgeon carries in his Lancet-Case with his Plaister-Box; and not portable are those that he doth not carry about him, but is oblig'd to keep at home; the former being appointed for the ready help which he daily administers to his Patients, and the others for greater Operations.

What are the Instruments which a Surgeon ought to have in his Plaister-Box?

These Instruments are a good pair of Sizzers, a Razor, an Incision-Knife streight and crooked, a Spatula, a greater Lancet to open Impostumes, and lesser for letting Blood. They likewise carry separately in very neat Lancet-Cases, a hollow Probe made of Silver or fine Steel; as also many other Probes, streight, crooked, folding, and of different thickness; a Pipe of Silver or fine Steel, to convey the cauterizing Button to a remote Part, without running the hazard of burning those that are near it; another Pipe or Tube serving instead of a Case for Needles, which have Eyes at one end for sowing; a Carlet, or thick triangular Needle; a small File; a Steel Instrument to cleanse the Teeth; a {6} Fleam; a pair of crooked Forceps to draw a Tooth; a Pelican; a Crow's Bill; several sorts of Raspatories; a Hook to hold up the Skin in cutting, &c.

What are the Instruments which a Surgeon ought to keep in his Repository to perform the greater Operations?

Some of them are peculiar to certain Operations, and others are common to all. The Instruments appropriated to particular Operations, are the Trepan for opening the Bones in the Head, or elsewhere: The Catheters or Probes for Men and Women afflicted with the Stone, or difficulty of making Water. Extractors, to lay hold on the Stone in Lithotomy, and to gather together the Gravel; large crooked Incision-Knives, and a Saw, to make Amputations of the Arms or Legs; great Needles with three Edges, to be used in making Setons; small Needles to couch Cataracts; other Needles; thin Plates and Buckles to close a Hair-Lip, &c.

May not the Salvatory be reckon'd among the portable Instruments?

Yes, because the Balsams, Ointments, and Plaisters contain'd therein, are means whereof the Surgeon makes use to restore Health.

* * * * *

CHAP. III.

Of Anatomy in general; and in particular of all the Parts whereof the Humane Body is compos'd.

What is Anatomy?

It is the Analysis or exact Division of all the Parts of a Body, to discover their Nature and Original.

What is requisite to be observ'd by a Surgeon before he goes about to dissect a Body?

Two things; viz. The external Structure of the Body, and the Proportion or Correspondence between the outward Parts, and those that are within.

Why so?

Because without this exterior and general Knowledge, the Surgeon wou'd be often mistaken in the Judgment he is to pass concerning a Dislocation or Wound, inasmuch as it is by the Deformity which he perceives in the Member, that he knows the Dislocation, as it is also by the means of the Correspondence which the outward Parts have with the inward, that he is enabled to draw any certain Consequences relating to a Wound, which penetrates into the Body.

What is a Part?

It is that whereof the whole Body is compos'd, and which partakes of a common Life or Sensation with it. {8}

How many sorts of Parts are there in a Humane Body?

We may well reckon up Fifteen distinct Parts, which are the Bone, the Cartilage, the Ligament, the Tendon, the Membrane, the Fibre, the Nerve, the Vein, the Artery, the Flesh, the Fat, the Skin, the Scarf-Skin, the Hair, and the

Nails.

What is a Bone?

It is the hardest and driest Part of the whole Body, and that which constitutes its principal Support.

What is a Cartilage or Gristle?

It is a yielding and supple Part, which partakes of the Nature of a Bone, and is always fasten'd to its Extremities, to mollifie and facilitate its Motion.

What is a Ligament?

It is a Membranous Contexture usually sticking to the Bones to contain them; as also sometimes to other Parts, to suspend, and retain them in their proper place.

What is a Tendon?

It is the Tail or Extremity of the Muscles, made by the re-union of all the Fibres of their Body, which serves to corroborate it in its Action, and to give Motion to the Part.

What is a Membrane?

It is a Nervous Part, the use whereof is to adorn and secure the Cavities of the Body on the inside, and to wrap up or cover the Parts.

What is a Fibre?

They are fleshy Lines of which the Body of a Muscle is compos'd.

What is a Nerve?

It is a long, white, and thin Body, consisting {9} of many Fibres, enclos'd within a double Tunick, and design'd to carry the Animal Spirits into all the Parts, to give them Sense and Motion.

What is an Artery?

It is a Canal compos'd of Four Coats, that carreyth with a kind of Beating or Pulse even to the very Extremity of the Parts, the Blood full of Spirits, which proceeds from the Heart, to distribute to them at the same time both Life and Nourishment.

What is a Vein?

It is a Canal made likewise of Four Tunicles, which receives the Arterial Blood, to carry it back to the Heart.

What is Flesh?

It is a Part which is form'd of Blood thicken'd by the natural Heat; and that constitutes the Body of a Muscle.

What is Fat?

It is a soft Body made of the Unctuous and Sulphurous part of the Blood.

What is the Derma or Skin?

It is a Net compos'd of Fibres, Veins, Arteries, Lymphatick Vessels and Nerves, which covers the whole Body to defend it from the Injuries of the Air, and to serve as a universal Emunctory: It is very thin in the Face, sticking close to the Flesh, and is pierc'd with an infinite number of imperceptible Pores, affording a Passage to insensible Transpiration.

What is the Epiderma, or Scarf-Skin?

It is a small fine Skin, transparent and insensible, having also innumerable Pores for the discharging of Sweat, and other Humours by {10} imperceptible Transpiration: It is extended over the whole inner Skin, to dull its too exquisite Sense, by covering the Extremities of the Nerves which are there terminated. It also renders the same Skin even and smooth, and so contributes very much to Beauty.

What is the Hair?

The Hairs are certain hollow Filaments planted in the Glandules of the Skin, from whence their Nourishment is deriv'd. They constitute the Ornament of some Parts, cover those which Modesty requires to be conceal'd, and defend others from the injury of the Weather.

What is a Nail?

The Nails are a Continuity of the Skin harden'd at the end of the Fingers, to strengthen and render them fit for Work.

* * * * *

CHAP. IV.

Of the general Division of a Humane Body.

How is the Humane Body divided before it is dissected, in order to Anatomical Demonstration?

Some Anatomists distinguish it into Similar and Dissimilar Parts, appropriating the former Denomination to all the simple Parts of the Body taken separately, as a Bone, a Vein, a Nerve, &c. but they attribute the Name of Dissimilar to all those Members that are compos'd of many Similar or Simple Parts together; such are the Arms, {11} Legs, Eyes, &c. wherein are contain'd all at once, Bones, Veins, Nerves, and other parts.

Others divide it into containing and contained Parts, the former enclosing the others, as the Skull includes the Brain, and the Breast the Lungs; whereas the contained Parts are shut up within others; as the Entrails within the Belly, the Brain within the Skull, &c.

Others again divide the whole Body into Spermatick and Sanguineous Parts; the former being those which are made at the time of Formation; and the latter all those that are grown afterward by the Nourishment of the Blood.

Are there not also other Methods of dividing the Humane Body?

Yes: Many Persons consider it as a Contexture of Bones, Flesh, Vessels and Entrails, which they explain in four several Treatises, whereof the first is call'd Osteology, for the Bones; the second Myology, for the Muscles; the third Angiology, for the Veins, Arteries and Nerves, which are the Vessels; and the fourth Splanchnology, for the Entrails.

But lastly, the most clear and perspicuous of all the Divisions of the Body of Man, is that which compares it to a Tree, whereof the Trunk is the Body, and the Branches are the Arms and Legs. The Body is divided into three Venters, or great Cavities, viz. the Upper, the Middle, and the Lower, which are the Head, the Breast, and the lower Belly. The Arms are distributed into the Arms properly so called, the Elbow and Hands; and the Legs in like manner into Thighs, Shanks, {12} and Feet: The Hands being also subdivided into the Carpus or Wrist, Metacarpium or Back of the Hand, and the Fingers; as the Feet into the Tarsus, Metatarsus, and Toes. This vision is at present follow'd in the Anatomical Schools.

* * * * *

CHAP. V.

Of the Skeleton.

Why is Anatomy usually begun with the Demonstration of the Skeleton, or Contexture of Bones?

Because the Bones serve for the Foundation Connexion, and Support of all other Parts of the Body.

What is the Skeleton?

It is a gathering together, or Conjunction of all the Bones of the Body almost in their Natural Situation.

From whence are the principal differences of the Bones derived?

They are taken from their Substance, Figure, Articulation, and Use.

How is all this to be understood?

First then, with respect to their Substance, there are some Bones harder than others; as those of the Legs compared with those of the Back-Bone. Again, in regard of their Figure, some are long, as those of the Arm; and others short, as those of the Metacarpium. Some are also broad, as those of the Skull and {13} Omoplat?or Shoulder-Blades; and others narrow, as the Ribbs. But with respect to their Articulation, some are joined by thick Heads, which are received into large Cavities, as the Huckle-Bones with those of the Hips; and others are united by the means of a simple Line, as the Chin-Bones. Lastly, with relation to their Use; some serve to support and carry the whole Body, as the Leg-Bones, and others are appointed to grind the Meat, as the Teeth; or else to form some Cavity, as the Skull-Bone, and those of the Ribs.

What are the Parts to be distinguished in the Bones?

They are the Body, the Ends, the Heads, the Neck, the Apophyses, the Epiphyses, the Condyli or Productions, the Cavities, the Supercilia or Lips, and the Ridges.

The Body is the greatest Part, and the middle of the Bone; the Ends are the two Extremities; the Heads are the great Protuberances at the Extremities; the Neck is that Part which lies immediately under the Head; the Apophyses or Processes are certain Bunches or Knobs at the Ends of the Bones, which constitute a Part of them; the Epiphyses are Bones added to the Extremities of other Bones; the Condyli or Productions are the small Elevations or Extuberances of the Bones; the Cavities are certain Holes or hollow places; the Supercilia or Lips are the Extremities of the Sides of a Cavity, which is at the End of a Bone; the Ridges are the prominent and saliant Parts in the length of the Body of the Bone. {14}

How are the Bones join'd together?

Two several ways, viz. by Articulation and Symphysis.

How many sorts of Articulations are there in the Bones?

There are generally two kinds, viz. Diarthrosis and Synarthrosis.

What is Diarthrosis?

Diarthrosis is a kind of Articulation which serves for sensible Motions.

How many kinds of Diarthroses, or great Motions are there?

There are Three, viz. Enarthrosis, Arthrodia, and Ginglymus.

Enarthrosis is a kind of Articulation which unites two Bones with a great Head on one side, and a large Cavity on the other; as the Head of the Thigh-Bone in the Cavity of the Ischion or Huckle-Bone.

Arthrodia is a sort of Articulation, by the means whereof two Bones are join'd together with a flat Head receiv'd into a Cavity of a small depth. Such is the Head of the Shoulder-Bone with the Cavity of the Omoplata or Shoulder-Blade; and that of the Twelfth Vertebra of the Back with the first of the Loins.

Ginglymus is a kind of Articulation which unites two Bones, each whereof hath at their Ends a Head and a Cavity, whereby they both receive and are received at the same time, such is the Articulation in the Bones of the Elbow and the Vertebr?

What is Synarthrosis?

Synarthrosis being opposite to Diarthrosis, is a {15} close or compacted Articulation, destitute of any sensible Motion.

How many sorts of Synarthroses, or close Articulations are there?

There are Three. viz. Sutura, Harmonia, and Gomphosis.

A Suture is that which joins together two Bones by a kind of Seam or Stitch, or by a Connexion of their Extremities dispos'd in form of a Saw, the Teeth whereof are reciprocally let one into another: Such are the Sutures of the Skull-Bones.

Harmonia is the uniting of two Bones by a simple Line; as the Bone of the Cheek with that of the Jaw.

Gomphosis is a kind of close Articulation, which unites two Bones after the manner of Nails or Wooden Pins fixt in the Holes made to receive them: Such is that of the Teeth in their Sockets.

What is Symphysis?

Symphysis is the uniting of two Bones by the interposition of a Medium, which ties them very streight together, being also threefold: Such is the Connexion of the Knee-Pan or Whirl-Bone of the Knee, and the Omoplata or Shoulder-Blade.

Are not these three kinds of Articulations or Symphyses distinguish'd one from another?

Yes; for tho' they are all made by the means of a third Body intervening, which joins them together; nevertheless every one of these various Bodies gives a different Denomination to its respective Articulation: Thus the Articulation which is caus'd by a Glutinous and {16} Cartilaginous Substance, is properly call'd Synchondrosis; as that of the Nose, Chin, Os Pubis, &c. But an Articulation which is made by a Ligament is termed Synncurosis, as that of the Knee-Pan. Lastly, that which is wrought by the means of Flesh, bears the Name of Syssarcosis; as the Jaw-Bones, the Os Hyoides, and the Omoplata or Shoulder-Blade.

Have the Bones any sense of Feeling or Motion?

They have neither; for their sense of Pain proceeds from nothing else but their Periostium, or the Membrane with which they are cover'd, and their Motion is perform'd only by the Muscles that draw them.

Doth the Marrow afford any Nutriment to the Bones?

No, all the Bones are nourish'd by the Blood, as the other Parts; but the Marrow is to the Bones what the Fat is to the Flesh; that is to say, it is a kind of Oil or Unctuous Substance, which moistens, and renders them less brittle.

Are all the Bones of the same Colour?

No, they follow the Temperament and Constitution of the Persons.

How many in number are the Bones of the Humane Skeleton?

There are two hundred and fifty usually reckon'd, viz. 61 in the Head, 67 in the Trunk or Chest, 62 in the Arms and Hands, and 60 in the Legs and Feet; but the true Number cannot be exactly determin'd, by reason that some Persons have more, and others fewer; for some have more Ossa Sesamoidea, Teeth and {17} Breast-Bones than others: Again, some have many indentings in the Lambdoidal Suture, and others have none at all.

Can you rehearse the Number of the Bones of the Head?

There are Fifteen in the Skull, and Forty six in the Face.

The Fifteen of the Skull are the Coronal for the fore-part of the Head; the Occipital for the hinder-part; the two Parietals for the upper-part and each side; the two Temporals for the Temples; the Os Sphenoides or Cuneiforme, which closeth the Basis or bottom of the Skull; the Os Ethmoides, or Cribriforme, situated at the Root of the Nose; and the four little Bones of the Ear on each side, viz. the Incus or Anvil; the Stapes or Stirrup; the Malleolus or Hammer; and the Orbiculare or Orbicular Bone.

Of the Forty six of the Face, Twenty seven are counted in the Upper-Jaw, viz. the two Zygomatick, or the two Bones of the Cheek-Knots; the two Lachrymal in the great Corners of the Eyes toward the Nose; the two Maxillar, that receive the Upper-Teeth, and which form part of the Palate of the Mouth, and the Orbits of the Eyes; the two Bones of the Nose; the two Palate-Bones which are at its end, and behind the Nostrils; the last being single is the Vomer, which makes the Division of the lower part of the Nostrils; and there are generally Sixteen Upper-Teeth. The Lower-Jaw contains Nineteen Bones, viz. sixteen Teeth; two Bones that receive them; and the Os Hyoides, which is single, and fix'd at the Root of the Tongue. {18}

How are the Teeth usually divided with respect to their Qualities?

Into Incisive or Cutters, Canine or Dog-Teeth, and Molar or Grinders: There are eight Incisive, and four Canine, which have only one single Root; as also twenty Molar, every one whereof hath one, two, or three Roots.

Can you recite the Number of the Bones of the Trunk or Chest?

There are generally thirty and three in the Spine or Chine-Bone of the Back, viz. seven Vertebra's in the Neck, twelve in the Back, five in the Legs, five, six, and sometimes seven in the Os Sacrum, three or four in the Coccyx, and two Cartilages at its end.

There are twenty nine in the Breast, viz. twenty four Ribs, two Clavicles or Channel-Bones and commonly three Bones in the Sternum. The Hip-Bones are likewise divided into three, viz. Ilion, Ischion and Os Pubis.

Do you know the Number of the Bones of the Arms?

There are thirty and one Bones in each Arm, that is to say, the Omoplata or Shoulder-Blade; the Humerus or Shoulder-Bone; the two Bones of the Elbow call'd Ulna, and Radius; eight little Bones in the Carpus or Wrist; five in the Metacarpium or Back of the Hand; and fourteen in the Fingers, three to every one except the Thumb, which hath only two.

Can you give us a List of the Bones of the Leg in their Order?

There are thirty Bones in each Leg, viz. the Femur or great Thigh-Bone, the Knee-Pan or {19} Whirl-Bone on the top of the Knee; the Tibia, greater Focile, or Shin-Bone; and the Perone or Fibula, or lesser Focile, which are the two associated Bones of the Leg; seven little Bones in the Tarsus; five in the Metatarsus; and fourteen in the Toes; that is to say, three to every one, except the great Toe, which hath only two.

Thus the Number of Bones of the Humane Skeleton amounts to two hundred and Fifty, without reckoning the Sesamoides, the Indentings of the Skull, and some others which are not always to be found.

* * * * *

CHAP. VI.

Of Myology, or the Anatomy of the Muscles of a Humane Body.

What is a Muscle?

It is the principal Organ or Instrument of Motion; or it is a Portion of Flesh, wherein there are Veins, Arteries, Nerves, and Fibres, and which is cover'd with a Membrane.

How many parts are there in a Muscle?

Three, viz. the Head, the Belly, and the Tail: The Head is that part thro' which the Nerve enters; the Belly is the Body or Middle of the Muscle; and the Tail is the Extremity, where all the Fibres of the Muscle are terminated to make the Tendon or String which is fasten'd to the Part whereto it gives Motion. {20}

Have all the Muscles their Fibres streight from the Head to the Tail?

No, some have them streight, others transverse, and others oblique or circular, according to the several Motions to which they are appropriated.

How many sorts of Muscles are there with respecting to their Action?

There are two different kinds, viz. the Antagonists and the Congenerate; the former are those that produce opposite Motions; as a Flexor and an Extensor, a Depressor and a Levator. The Congenerate are those that contribute to one and the same Action; as when there are two Flexors or two Extensors, and then one supplies the defect of the other; whereas when one of the Antagonist Muscles is cut, the other becomes useless, and void of Action.

How is the Action of a Muscle perform'd?

It is done by Contraction and Extension; the former causeth the Antagonist to swell, and the other compels it to stretch forth in length.

What is Aponeurosis?

It is the continuity of the Fibres of a Tendon which makes a Connexion that serves to strengthen the Muscle in its Motion.

* * * * *

CHAP VII.

Of the Myology, or Anatomy of the Muscles of the Head.

How many Muscles are there appointed to move the Head, and which be they?

The Head is mov'd by the means of fourteen Muscles, seven on each side; of these, two serve to depress it, eight to lift it up, and four to turn it round about.

The two Depressors are call'd Sternoclinomastoidei; they take their Rise in the Sternum, at the Clavicles, and proceed obliquely to join the Apophysis Mastoides.

Of the four Elevators on each side the first is the Splenius, which begins at the five Vertebr?of the Back and the three lower ones of the Neck, and ascending obliquely, cleaves to the hinder part of the Head. The second, named Complexus or Trigeminus, having its beginning as the Splenius, sticks in like manner to the hinder part of the Head, and they form together a figure resembling that of S. Andrew's Cross. The third is the Rectus Major, which proceeding from the second Vertebra of the Neck, shoots forward to join the hinder part of the Head. The fourth is the Rectus Minor, which begins at the first Vertebra of the Neck, and ends likewise in the hinder part of the Head.

The two Muscles on each side, which move the Head circularly, are the Obliquus Major and {22} Minor; the greater Oblique taking its rise from the second Vertebra of the Neck, goes to meet the first; but the lesser Oblique hath its Origine in the hinder part of the Head, and proceeds to join the other obliquely in the first Vertebra.

How many Muscles are there in the Lower-Jaw, and which be they?

The Lower-Jaw hath twelve Muscles which cause it to move; that is to say, six on each side, whereof four serve to close and two to open it.

The first of the Openers is the Latus, which beginning at the top of the Sternum, Clavicle, and Acromion, cleaves on the outside to the bottom of the Lower-Jaw-Bone. The second of the Openers is the Digastricus, which takes its rise in a Fissure lying between the Occipital Bone and the Apophysis Mastoides, from whence it passeth to the bottom of the Chin on the inside.

The first of the Shutters is the Crotaphites or Temporal Muscle, which hath its Origine at the bottom, and on the side of the Os Coronale, the Os Parietale, and the Os Petrosum, from whence it is extended till it cleaves to the Apophysis Coronoides of the Lower-Jaw, after having passed above the Apophysis of the Zygoma: Its Fibres are spread from the Circumference to the Center, and it is covered again with the Pericranium, which renders its Wounds very dangerous; so that the least Incisions as can be, ought to be made therein.

The second is the Pterygoideus or Aliformis Externus, whose rise is in the Apophysis Pterygoides, from whence it sets forward till it stick between the Condylus and the Coronal of the Lower-Jaw.

The third is the Masseter, which hath two {23} Sources or Beginnings, and as many Insertions; the first Source thereof is at the Cheek-Knot or Ball of the Cheek, and the second at the lower part of the Zygoma. The first Insertion is at the outer Corner of the Jaw, and the second in the middle part, by that means forming the Figure of the Letter X.

The fourth is the Pterygoideus or Aliformis Internus, which hath its beginning in the Apophysis Pterygoides, and is terminated in the inner Corner of the Jaw; so that Mastication or Chewing is perform'd by the means of these four Muscles.

How many Muscles are there in the Face, and which be they?

There are two for the Forehead, call'd Frontal, whose Origine is in the upper part of the Head, from whence they descend by streight Fibres, until they are fasten'd in the Skin of the Forehead near the Eye-Brows, where they are re-united: Their Action or Office is to draw the Skin of the Forehead upward, whereto they stick very close.

There are also two others call'd Occipital, which have their Beginning in the same place with the preceeding, but they descend backward, and cleave to the Skin of the hinder part of the Head, which they draw upward.

There are two Muscles to each Eye-Lid, one whereof is termed the Attollens or Elevator and the other the Depressor. The Elevator takes its rise in the bottom of the Orbit of the Eye, and is fastned by a large Aponeurosis to the edge of the upper Eye-Lid. The Shutter or Depressor, call'd also the Orbicular, hath its Origine in the great Canthus, or Corner of the Eye, passeth over the {24} Eye-Lid upward, and is join'd to the lesser Corner of the same Eye, being extended along its whole Compass.

The Eyes have each six Muscles, viz. four Recti and two Obliqui; the Recti or streight Muscles are the Elevator, the Depressor, the Adductor, and the Abductor. The first of these call'd Elevator, or Superbus, draws the Eye upward, as it is pull'd downward by the Depressor or Humilis; the Adductor or Bibitorius draws it toward the Nose, and the Abductor or Indignarorius toward the Shoulder: All these small Muscles have their Originals and Insertions in the bottom of the Orbit through which the Optick Nerve passeth, and are terminated in the Corneous Tunicle, by a very large Tendon.

The first of the Oblique ones is term'd the Obliquus Major, and the other Obliquus Minor, because they draw the Eye obliquely. These Muscles cause Children to squint when they do not act together. The Obliquus Minor is fasten'd at the outward part of the Orbit near the great Corner, and draws the Eye obliquely toward the Nose: But the Obliquus Major is fixt in the inner part of the Orbit, and ascends along the Bone to the upper part of the great Corner, where its Tendon passeth thro' a small Cartilage nam'd Trochlea, and is inserted in the little Corner with the lesser Obliquus Minor, to draw the Eye obliquely toward the lesser Corner.

The Ear, altho' not usually endu'd with any sensible Motion, nevertheless hath four Muscles, viz. one above, and three behind; the first being situated over the Temporal, and fasten'd to the Ear to draw it upward: The three others have {25} their beginning in the Mammillary Apophysis, and are terminated in the Root of the Ear, to draw it backward.

There are also three Muscles in the inner part of the Ear, whereof the external belonging to the Malleus or Hammer lies under the exterior part of the Bony Passage which reacheth from the Ear to the Palate of the Mouth, being fixt in a very oblique Sinuosity which is made immediately above the Bone that bears the Furrow, into which is let the Skin of the Tympanum or Drum. The internal Muscle lies hid in a Bony Semi-Canal, in the Os Petrosum; one part of which Semi-Canal is without the Drum, and clos'd on the top with a Passage that leads from the Ear into the Palate. But the other part within the Drum advanceth to the Fenestra Ovalis, and is inserted in the hinder part of the Handle of the Malleus. The Muscle of the Stapes or Stirrup is also hid in a Bony Tube, almost at the bottom of the Drum, and fixt in the Head of the Stapes.

The Nose hath seven Muscles, that is to say, one common and six proper; the common constitutes part of the orbicular Muscle of the Lips, and draws the Nose downward with the Lip. Of the six proper Muscles of the Nose, four serve to dilate it, being situated on the outside, and two to contract it, which are placed in the inside.

The two first Dilatators of a Pyramidal Figure, take their rise in the Suture of the Forehead, and are fasten'd by a large Filament to the Al?of the Nose. The two other Dilatators resembling a Myrtle-Leaf have their Source in {26} the Bone of the Nose, and are inserted in the middle of the Ala.

The two Restrictors are Membranous, beginning in the internal part of the Bone of the Nose and adhering to the inner Ala of the Nostril.

The Lips have thirteen Muscles, viz. eight proper, and five common: Of the proper there are four for the Upper-Lip, and as many for the Lower: with two common for each, and the odd one.

The first of the proper of the Upper-Lip bears the Name of the Incisivus, its Origine being in the Jaw, in the place of the Incisive Teeth and its Insertion is in the Upper-Lip.

The second is the Triangulis, Antagonist to the former; its Rise is on the outside, at the bottom of the Lower-Jaw; and it is implanted in the Upper-Lip, near the Corner of the Mouth.

The third being the Quadratus, springs from the bottom of the Chin before, and cleaves to the edge of the Lower-Lip.

The fourth is the Caninus, Antagonist to the Quadratus, beginning in the Upper-Jaw-Bone and being terminated in the Lower-Lip near the Corner of the Mouth.

The first of the common is the Zygomaticus, the Origine whereof is in the Zygoma and its Insertion in the Corner of the Mouth, to draw it toward the Ears; so that it is the Muscle which acts when we laugh.

The second of the common is the Buccinator or Trumpeter, which is swell'd when one sounds a Trumpet. It hath its rise at the Root of the Molar Teeth of both the Jaws, and is extended quite round about the Lips. {27}

The odd Muscle, or the thirteenth in number, is the Orbicular, which makes a Sphincter round about the Lips to close or shut them up.

The Uvula or Palate of the Mouth hath four Muscles, whereof the two first are the Peristaphylini Externi, taking their rise from the Upper-Jaw, above the Left Molar Tooth, and being ty'd to the Palate by a thin Tendon.

The two others are the Peristaphylini Interni, which have their beginning in the Apophysis Pterygoides on the inside, and likewise stick to the Palate.

The Tongue, altho' all over Musculous and Fibrous, yet doth not cease to have its peculiar Muscles, which are eight in Number.

The first of these is call'd Genioglossus, taking its rise in the lower part of the Chin, from whence it is extended till it cleave to the Root of the Tongue before, to cause it to go out of the Mouth.

The second is term'd Styloglossus, its Rise being in the Apophysis Styloides, from whence it passeth to the side above the Tongue, to lift it up.

The third bearing the Name of Basiglossus, commenceth in the Basis or Root of the Os Hyoides, and thence insinuates it self into the Root of the Tongue, to draw it back to the bottom of the Mouth.

The fourth is the Ceratoglossus, deriving its Original from the Horn of the Os Hyoides, and cleaving to the side of the Tongue to draw it on one side: The Action of these Muscles of both sides together, causeth an Orbicular Motion in the Tongue. To these some add a fifth {28} Pair of Muscles, call'd Myloglossus, which serves to draw it obliquely upward.

What is the Action of the Os Hyoides in the Throat, and how many Muscles hath it?

The use of the Os Hyoides is to consolidate the Root of the Tongue; and it hath five Muscles on each side, which keep it as it were hung up.

The first of these, call'd the Geniohyoideus hath its beginning in the Chin on the inside, and adheres to the top of the Os Hyoides, which it draws upward.

The second is the Mylohyoideus, whose Origine is in the inner side of the Jaw, from whence it cleaves side-ways to the Root of the Os Hyoides, which it draws upward, and to one side.

The third is the Stylohyoideus, which after it hath taken its rise in the Apophysis Styloides, is fasten'd to the Horn of the Os Hyoides, to draw it toward the side.

The fourth is the Coracohyoideus, which springing up from the Apophysis Coracoides of the Omoplata, cleaves to the Root and side of the Os Hyoides, to draw it downward and to the side.

The fifth is the Sternomohyoideus, that hath its beginning in the Bone of the Sternum on the inside and is inserted in the Root of the Os Hyoides, which it draws downward.

How many Muscles hath the Larynx?

There are fourteen, viz. four Common, and ten Proper. The first Pair of the Common is the Sternothyroideus or Bronchycus, which proceeding from the inside, and the top of the Sternum, ascends along the Cartilages of the Wind-Pipe, and is terminated in the bottom of the {29} Scutiformis or Buckler-like Cartilage, which it draws downward. The second is the Hyothyroideus, which ariseth from the Root of the Os Hyoides, and is inserted in that of the Scutiforme. This Muscle serves to lift up the Larynx, as also to dilate the bottom of the Scutiformis, and to close its top.

The first Pair of the Proper is the Cricothyroideus Anticus, which deriving its Original from the hinder and upper part of the Cricoides, or Ring-like Cartilage, is fixt in the upper and lateral part of the Scutiformis, to close or shut it up.

The second is the Thyroides.

The third is the Cricoarytenoideus Lateralis, which proceeds from the side of the Cricoides within, and is fasten'd to the bottom and side of the Arytenoides, which it removes to dilate the Mouth of the Larynx.

The fourth is the Thyroarytenoideus, which arising from the fore-part on the inside of the Scutiformis, is terminated on the side of the Arytenoides, to close the Orifice of the Larynx.

The fifth is the Arytenoideus, which having its Source in that place where the Cricoides is united to the Arytenoides is inserted in its upper and lateral part, to close the Larynx.

How many Muscles hath the Pharynx?

It hath seven, the first whereof is the Oesophagieus, which takes its rise from the side of the Scutiformis or Buckler-like Cartilage, and passing behind the Oesophagus or Gullet, is fasten'd to the other side of the Cartilage. It thrusts the Meat down by locking up the Pharynx as a Sphincter.

The second named Stylopharingus, springs from within the Acute Apophysis of the Os Sphenoides, or Cuneiforme, and is inserted obliquely {30} in the side of the Pharynx, which it dilates by drawing it upward.

The third, call'd Sphenopharyngus, proceeds from the Apophysis Styliformis, and is terminated in the side of the Pharynx, which it dilates by drawing its sides.

The fourth Pair is the Cephalopharyngus which ariseth from the articulation of the Head with the first Vertebra, and closeth the Larynx.

How many Muscles are there in the Neck, and which be they?

There are four Muscles in the Neck on each side, viz. two Flexors, and two Extensors. The Flexors are the Scalenus and the Rectus or Longus; and the Extenders are the Spinatus and the Transversalis.

The Scalenus or Triangularis hath two remote Sources, viz. one in the first Rib, and the other in the Clavicle, and is fasten'd to the third and fourth Vertebra of the Neck.

The Rectus or Longus begins in the side of the four upper Vertebra's of the Back, and is join'd to the upper Vertebra's of the Neck, and the hinder part of the Head.

The Spinatus hath its Origine in the fourth and fifth upper Vertebra's of the Back, and is fasten'd to all the six lower Vertebra's of the Neck.

The Transversalis springs forth out of the upper Vertebra's of the Back, and cleaves to the Extremity of the four Vertebra's of the Neck.

* * * * *

{31}

CHAP. VIII.

Of the Myology or Anatomy of the Muscles of the Chest; or of the Breast

Belly, and Back.

How many Muscles are there in the Breast, and which be they?

The Breast hath fifty seven Muscles, that is to say, thirty that serve to dilate it, twenty six whose Office is to contract it, and the Diaphragm or Midriff, which partakes of both Actions.

The thirty which dilate the Breast are equally plac'd to the number of Fifteen, viz. the Subclavius, the Serratus Major Anticus, the two Serrati Postici, and the eleven external Intercostals.

The twenty six which contract the Breast are likewise equally rank'd to the Number of thirteen on each side, viz. the Triangularis, the Sacrolumbus, and eleven internal Intercostals.

The Subclavian takes up the whole space between the Clavicle and the first Rib: Its Original being in the internal and lower part of the Clavicula, and its insertion in the upper part of the first Rib.

The Serratus Major is a large Muscle having seven or eight Indentings or Jaggs. It takes its rise in the interior Basis of the Omoplata or Shoulder-Blade, and its Jaggings are inserted in {32} the five lower true Ribs, as also in the two upper spurious Ribs.

The Serratus Posticus Superior, begins with a large Aponeurosis in the Apophyses of the three lower Vertebr?of the Neck, and of the first of those of the Back; then passing under the Rhomboid, it is join'd obliquely by four Indentings to the four upper Ribs.

The Serratus Posticus Inferior, commences in like manner with a large Aponeurosis in the Apophyses of the three lower Vertebra's of the Back, and of the first of those of the Loins, and is afterwards fasten'd by four Digitations to the four lower Ribs.

The eleven External Intercostal Muscles are situated in the spaces between the twelve Ribs passing obliquely and on the outside from the back part to the fore part. They take their rise below the Upper Rib, and have their

Insertion above the lower Rib.

The Triangularis is the first of those that contract the Breast, and possesseth the inward part of the Sternum: Its Original is in its lower part, and its Insertion in the top of the Cartilages of the two upper Ribs.

The Sacrolumbus hath its Source in the hinder part of the Os Sacrum, as also in the Vertebra's of the Loins, and ascending from thence, insinuates it self into the hinder part of the Ribs, to every one of which it imparts two Tendons, one whereof sticks on the outside, and the other on the inside. This Muscle is fleshy within, and fibrous without.

The Eleven Internal Intercostals, contrary to the External, derive their Original from the {33} top of every lower Rib, and ascend obliquely from the back-part to the fore-part, till they are join'd to the lower Lip of every upper Rib: Thus these Internal Muscles, with the External, form, by the opposition of their Fibres, a Figure resembling a Burgundian Cross.

The Diaphragm or Midriff is esteem'd as the fifty seventh Muscle of the Breast, and serves as well for its dilatation as contraction. It separates the Thorax or Chest from the lower Belly, and is tied circularly to all the Extremities of the Bastard Ribs, immediately under the Xiphoides, or Sword-like Cartilage.

Modern Anatomists have discover'd that the Diaphragm is compos'd of two Muscles, viz. one Upper, and the other Lower; so that the Upper cleaves to the Extremities of the Spurious Ribs, and is terminated in a flat Tendon in the middle, which hath been always taken for its Nervous part. The Lower begins with two Productions, the longest whereof being on the right side, ariseth from the three upper Vertebra's of the Loins, and the other on the Left from the two Vertebra's of the Back, till it is lost in the Aponeurosis of the Upper Muscle.

How many Muscles are there in the Back and the Loins, and which be they?

There are three in each side, viz. one for Flection, and the other for Extension.

The Triangularis is the Flexor, taking its rise in the hinder part of the Rib of the Os Ilion, and the inner part of the Os Sacrum, in passing from whence it is joined to the last of the {34} Bastard Ribs, and to the transverse Productions of the Vertebra's of the Loins.

The Extensors are the Sacer, and the Semi-spinatus, which make the Waste streight, and are so interwoven along the Back-Bone, that one would imagine that there were as many Pairs of Muscles as Vertebra's, affording Tendons to all.

The Sacer springs from behind the Os Sacrum, as also from the hinder and upper Extremity of the Os Ilium, and is inserted in the Spines of the Vertebra's of the Loins and Back.

The Semi-spinatus hath its Source in the Spines of the Os Sacrum, and is join'd to all the transverse Productions of the Vertebra's from the Back to the Neck, being exactly situated between the Sacer and the Sacrolumbus.

* * * * *

CHAP. IX.

Of the Myology, or Anatomy of the Muscles of the lower Belly.

How many Muscles are there in the lower Belly, and which be they?

There are generally ten, five on each side, that is to say, two Obliqui, one ascending, and the other descending; one Transversus, one Rectus, and two Pyramidal, of which last, nevertheless, there is sometimes only one, and sometimes none at all. {35}

The Obliquus Descendens, which is the first, hath its Original by digitation in the sixth and seventh of the true Ribs, in all the spurious Ribs, and in the transverse Apophyses of the Vertebra's of the Loins, and comes near to the Serratus Major Anticus of the Breast; from whence it proceeds to the external Rib of the Os Ilion, and is terminated by a large Aponeurosis in the Linea Alba or White Line, which separates the Muscles that are on each side of the Abdomen or lower Belly.

The Obliquus Ascendens ariseth from its Source in the upper part of the Os Pubis, and in the Ridge of the Hip-Bone, till it cleaves to the Apophyses of the Vertebra's of the Loins in the Extremities of all the Ribs, and in the Xiphoides or Sword-like Cartilage, and is terminated in the White Line by a large Aponeurosis.

The Rectus being situated between the Aponeuroses of the Obliquus, takes its rise in the Cartilages of the Ribs, in the Xiphoides and the Sternum, and enters into the Os Pubis, having many nervous parts to corroborate it in its length.

The Transversus having its beginning in the transverse Apophyses of the Vertebra's of the Loins, is fasten'd to the internal Rib of the Os Ilium, and within the Cartilages of the lower Ribs, and is terminated by a large Aponeurosis in the Linea Alba, passing over the Rectus, and sticking to the Peritoneum.

The Oblique Muscles, and the Transverse, have Holes toward the Groin, to give Passage to the Spermatick Vessels of Men, and to a round {36} ligament of the Matrix in Women; so that Ruptures or Burstenness happen through these parts in both Sexes, although the Holes of these three Muscles are not situated one over-against another.

The Pyramidal, so named by reason of its Figure, is situated in the lower Tendon of the Rectus, its Origine being in the upper and external part of the Os Pubis; but it is terminated in the White Line, three Fingers breadth above the Pubes, and sometimes even in the Navel itself. These Muscles are not found in all Bodies for there are sometimes two, sometimes only one, and sometimes none.

The use of the Muscles of the lower Belly is to compress all the contain'd parts, in order to assist them in expelling the Excrements.

How many Muscles are there in the Testicles?

They have each of them one, call'd Cremaster; this Muscle takes its rise from the Ligaments of the Os Pubis, and by the dilatation of its Tendon covers the

Testicle, which it draws upward.

How many Muscles hath the Penis?

It hath two Pair, viz. the Erectores or Directores, and the Dilatantes: The Erectores arise from the internal part of the Os Ischion, under the beginning of the Corpora Cavernosa, where they are inserted, and retake their Fibres in their Membranes. The Dilatantes or Acceleratores have their Source in the Sphincter of the Anus and slipping from thence obliquely under the Ureter, are join'd to the Membrane of the Nervous Bodies.

How many Muscles are there in the Clitoris? {37}

It hath two Erectors which spring forth from the Protuberance of the Os Ischion, and are inserted in the Nervous Bodies of the Clitoris. There are also two others suppos'd to be its Elevators, which proceed from the Sphincter of the Anus, and are terminated in the Clitoris.

How many Muscles are there in the Anus?

There are three, viz. the Sphincter, and two Levatores. The Sphincter is two Fingers broad, to open and close the Rectum. This Muscle being double, is fasten'd in the fore-part to the Penis in Men, and to the Neck of the Matrix in Women, as also behind to the Coccyx, and laterally to the Ligaments of the Os Sacrum, and the Hips.

The two Levatores arise from the inner and lateral part of the Os Ischion, and are fasten'd to the Sphincter of the Anus, to lift it up after the expulsion of the Excrements.

The Bladder hath also a Sphincter Muscle to open and shut its Orifice.

* * * * *

CHAP. X.

Of the Muscles of the Omoplat? or Shoulder-Blades, Arms, and Hands.

How many ways doth the Omoplata or Shoulder-Blade move, and what are its Muscles?

The Omoplata moves upward, downward, forward, and backward, by the means of four proper Muscles, which are the Trapezius, the {38} Rhomboides, the proper Levator, and the lesser Pectoral, or Serratus Minor Anticus.

The Trapezius or Cucullaris hath its beginning in the back part of the Occiput, or hinder part of the Head, in the Spines of the six lower Vertebra's of the Neck, and of the nine upper of the Back, in passing from whence it is implanted in the Spine of the Omoplata or Shoulder-Blade, and the external part of the Clavicula, as far as the Acromion. This Muscle produceth many Motions by reason of its different Fibres, drawing the Shoulder-Blade obliquely upward, downward, and forward.

The Rhomboides is situated over the Trapezius, its rise being in the Apophyses of the three lower Vertebra's of the Neck, and of the three upper of the Back, but it is afterward join'd to the whole Basis or Root of the Omoplata, which it draws backward.

The proper Levator commenceth in the Transverse Apophyses of the four first Vertebra's of the Neck, by different Progressions, but is afterward re-united, and inserted in the upper Corner of the Omoplata, which it draws upward.

The lesser Pectoral, or Serratus Minor Anticus, is situated under the great Pectoral, its rise being by Digitation or Indenting in the second, third, and fourth of the upper Ribs, and its Insertion in the Apophysis Coracoides of the Shoulder-Blade, which it draws forward.

How many Motions are there in the Humerus, or Arm; which be they, and what are its Muscles? {39}

The Arm performs all sorts of Motions by the help of nine Muscles: For it is lifted up by the Deltoides and the Infra-Spinatus; it is depress'd by the Largissimus, and the Rotundus Major; it is drawn forward by the Pectoralis Major, and the Coracoideus; it is drawn backward by the Infra-Spinatus, and the Rotundus Minor. It is drawn near the Ribs by the Subscapularis, and its circular Motion is performed when all these Muscles act together successively.

The Deltoides or Triangular hath its beginning in the whole Spine of the Omoplata, the Acromion, and half the Clavicula, and by its point cleaves with a strong Tendon to the middle of the Arm.

The Infra-Spinatus takes its rise in the Cavity that lies above the Spine of the Omoplata, which it fills, passing over the Acromion, until it is join'd to the Neck of the Shoulder-Bone, which it surrounds with a large Tendon.

The Largissimus, otherwise call'd Ani-scalptor, covers almost the whole Back, proceeding from a large and Nervous Stock, in the third and fourth lower Vertebra of the Back, the five Vertebra's of the Loins, the Spine of the Os Sacrum, the hinder part of the Lip of the Hip-Bone, and the external part of the lower Bastard-Ribs, in passing from whence it insinuates it self into the lower Corner of the Omoplata, as also into the upper and inner part of the Humerus.

The Rotundus Major, or Teres Major, having its Origin in the external Cavity of the lower Corner of the Omoplata, is confounded with the Largissimus, and adheres with it by the same {40} Tendon to the upper and inner part of the Humerus, a little below the Head.

The greater Pectoral hath its Source in half the Clavicula, on the side of the Sternum; covers the fore-part of the Breast, and is fasten'd by a short, broad, and nervous Tendon, to the top of the Shoulder-Bone, on the inside, between the Biceps and the Deltoides.

The Coracoideus or Coracobrachyus, beginning in the Apophysis Coracoides of the Omoplata or Shoulder-Blade, adheres to the middle of the Arm on the inside, which with the Pectoral it draws forward.

The Infra-Spinatus fills the Cavity which lies below the Spine of the Omoplata, its Origine being in the lower Rib of the Omoplata, from whence it passeth between the Spine and the Rotundus Minor, to cleave to the Neck of the Shoulder-Bone, which it embraceth, and draws backward.

The Rotundus Minor, or Teres Minor, proceeds from the lower Rib of the Omoplata, and adheres to the Neck of the Shoulder-Bone with the Infra-Spinatus to draw it in like manner backward.

The Sub-scapularis or Immersus is situated entirely under the Omaplata, proceeding from the internal Lip of the Basis or Root of the same Omoplata, and being terminated in the Neck of the Arm-Bone, which it causeth to lie close to the Ribs.

How many Motions are there in the Cubitus or Elbow, and what are its Muscles?

The Cubitus or Ulna is endu'd with two sorts of Motions, viz. that of Flection and that of {41} Extension, the former being perform'd by the help of two Muscles, that is to say, the Biceps, and the Brachius Internus; and the later by eight others, which are the Longus, the Brevis, the Brachius Externus, and the Anconeus.

The Biceps is a Muscle with two Heads, one whereof proceeds from the Apophysis Coracoides, and the other from the Cartilaginous edge of the Glenoid Cavity of the Omoplata or Shoulder-Blade: These two Heads descend along the fore-part of the Arm, and are united in one and the same Body, from whence springs forth a Ligament, which is inserted in a tuberosity situated in the upper and fore-part of the Radius.

The Brachius Internus is a small fleshy Muscle, lying hid under the Biceps, which takes its rise in the upper and fore-part of the Humerus, and is implanted in the upper and inner-part of the Radius, to bend the Elbow with the Biceps.

The first of the four Extenders is the Longus having two Sources, viz. one situated in the lower Rib of the Omoplata, near its Neck, and the other descending to the hinder-part of the Arm, till it is tyed to the Olecranum or Ancon, by a strong Aponeurosis, which is common thereto, with the Brevis, and the Brachius Externus.

The Brevis or short Muscle of the Elbow arising from the hinder and upper-part of the Humerus, is fasten'd to the Olecranum with the Longus.

The Brachius Externus is a fleshy Muscle which proceeds from the hinder part of the {42} Humerus, and adheres to the Olecranum with the Brevis and the Longus.

The Anconeus or Cubitalis being situated behind the Fold of the Cubitus, is the least Muscle of all; it springs from the Extremity of the Arm-Bone, at the end of the Brevis and the Longus, and in descending is inserted between the Radius and the Cubitus or Ulna, three or four Fingers breadth below the Olecranum.

How many Muscles hath the Radius, and which are its Motions?

The Radius is endu'd with a twofold Motion by the means of four Muscles: Of these the Rotundus and Quadratus cause that of Pronation, as the Longus and the Brevis that of Supination.

The Pronator Superior Rotundus, or round Muscle of the Radius, commenceth from the inner Apophysis of the Shoulder-Bone, in a very fleshy Stock, and is terminated obliquely by a Membranous Tendon in the middle and exterior part of the Radius.

The Pronator Inferior Quadratus, springing forth from the bottom and inside of the Cubitus, is fixt in the lower and outward part of the Radius by a Tail as large as its Head. This Muscle lying hid under the others near the Wrist, is that which jointly with the Rotundus, turns the Arm with the Palm of the Hand downward, which is the Motion of Pronation.

The Longus is the first of the Supinators, whose Origine is three or four Fingers breadth above the external Apophysis of the Arm-Bone; from whence it passeth along the Radius, and cleaves to the inner-part of its lower Apophysis. {43}

The Brevis, or the second of the Spinators arising from the lower part of the Inferior Condylus, and the external of the Humerus, is twisted round about the Radius, going forward from the hinder-part till it is united to its upper and forepart. This Muscle, with the Longus, serves to turn the Arm and the Palm of the Hand upward, and produceth the Motion of Supination.

How many sorts of Motions belong to the Wrist, and what are its Muscles?

Two several Motions are perform'd by the Wrist, viz. one of Flection, and the other of Extension, three Muscles being appropriated to the former, and as many to the later: But it ought to be observed, that a strong Ligament, call'd the Annular, appears here, which, surrounding all the Tendons of the Muscles as it were a Bracelet, holds them together, and elsewhere serves to unite the two Bones of the Elbow. The three Flexors or Bending Muscles of the Wrist are the Cubit 鶲 s Internus, the Radius Internus, and the Palmaris.

The Cubitus Internus derives its Original from the part of the Arm-Bone, passeth under the Annular Ligament, and is ty'd by a thick Tendon to the small Bone of the Wrist, which is plac'd above the others.

The Radi 鶲 s Internus proceeds from the same place with the Cubit 鶲 s, and is fasten'd to the first Wrist-Bone which supports the Thumb. It lies along the Radius, and passeth under the Annular Ligament.

The Palmaris is reckon'd among the Flexors of the Wrist, although situated in the Palm of the Hand. It ariseth from the inner Process or Knob {44} of the Arm-Bone, and is united by a large Tendon to the first Phalanges of the Fingers, slipping under the Transverse or Annular Ligament and sticking under the Skin of the Palm of the Hand.

The three extending Muscles of the Wrist are the Cubitus Externus, and the Radius Externus or the Longus, and the Brevis.

The Cubitus Externus taking its rise from the hinder-part of the Elbow, passeth under the Annular Ligament, and adheres to the upper and outward-part of the Bone of the Metacarpus that stayeth the little Finger.

The Radius Externus, or the Longus, having its Origine in the edge of the lower part of the Arm-Bone, slides from thence along the Radius on the outside, extends it self under the Annular Ligament, and cleaves to the Wrist-Bone, which stayeth the Fore-Finger.

The Brevis or short Muscle of the Wrist springs from the lower part of the same Edge; afterwards it runs along the Radius, passeth under the Annular Ligament, and is terminated in the Bone of the Carpus or Wrist, which stayeth the Middle Finger. But we must take notice, that besides these six Muscles, there is also a square piece of Flesh under the Palmaris, which seems to arise from the Thenar, and sticks to the eighth Wrist-Bone. It is supposed that this Musculous piece of Flesh serves with the Hypothenar of the little Finger, to make that which is call'd Diogenes's Cup.

How many Motions are there in the Fingers, and what are their Muscles? {45}

The Fingers are bent, extended, and turn'd from one side to the other by the means of twenty-three Muscles, whereof ten are proper, and thirteen common: The former are those that serve all the Fingers in general, and the other those that are particularly serviceable to some of them: The Common are the Sublimis, the Profundus, the common Extensor, the four Lumbricales, and the six Interossei.

The Sublimis or Perforatus, arising from the internal part of the lower Process of the Humerus or Shoulder-Bone is divided into four Tendons, which run below the Annular Ligament of the Wrist, and are inserted in the second Phalanx of the Bones of the four Fingers, after having stuck in passing to those of the first Phalanx, to help to bend it. It is also observed that every one of these Tendons hath a small cleft in its length, to let in the Tendons of the Profundus.

The Profundus or Perforans lies under the Sublimis, deriving its Original from the top of the Cubitus and Radius. It creeps along these two Bones, and is divided into four Tendons, which pass under the Annular Ligament, and slip into the Fissures of the Tendons of the Sublimis, to adhere to the third Phalanx of the Fingers, which they bend with the Sublimis: So that these two Muscles make together the bending of the Fingers.

The Extensor Magnus is that which extends the four Fingers. It springs from the external and lower Process of the Arm-Bone, and is divided into four flat Tendons, which pass under the Annular Ligament, and cleave {46} to the second and third Phalanx of the Fingers.

The four Lumbricales or Vermiculares are in the Palm of the Hand, to draw the Fingers to the Thumb: They proceed from the Tendons of the Profundus, and the Annular Ligament, extend themselves along the sides of the Fingers and are inserted in their second Articulation, to cause the drawing toward the Thumb.

The three Interossei Interni, and the three Externi, are situated between the four Bones of the Metacarpium, as well on the inside of the Hand as without: They have their beginning in the Intervals or Spaces between the Bones of the Metacarpium, are united with the Lumbrical, and fixt in the last Articulation of the Bones of the Fingers, to produce the Motion of drawing back or removing from the Thumb.

The Thumb is mov'd by five particular Muscles; one whereof serves to bend it, two to extend it, one to remove it from the Fingers, and another to draw it to them.

The Flexor of the Thumb takes its rise from the upper and inner part of the Radius, passes under the Annular Ligament, as also under the Thenar, and adheres to the first and second Bones of the same Thumb to bend it.

The two Extensors of the Thumb are the Longior and the Brevior: The former proceeding from the upper and outward part of the Cubitus, ascends above the Radius, and is ty'd with a forked Tendon to the second Bone of the Thumb. The Brevior hath the same Origin with the Longior, keeps the same Track, passes under the Annular Ligament, and is terminated in the third Thumb-Bone. {47}

The Thenar removes the Thumb from the Fingers, and forms that part which is call'd the Mount of Venus: It hath its Source in the first Bone of the Carpus or Wrist, and the Annular Ligament, and is inserted in its second Bone.

The Antithenar draws the Thumb to the other Fingers, having its Origine in the Bone of the Metacarpus, that stayeth the middle Finger, and its Insertion is in the first Bone of the Thumb.

The Muscle which serves to extend the Fore-Finger, is call'd Indicator: It proceeds from the middle and outer part of the Cubitus, and is fixt by a double Tendon in the second Articulation of the Fore-Finger, as also in the Tendon of the great Extensor of the Fingers.

That which draws the Fore-Finger to the Thumb is term'd Adductor: It commenceth in the fore-part of the first Thumb-Bone, and is terminated in the Bones of the Fore-Finger.

That which removes the Fore-Finger from the Thumb is known by the Name of Abductor, which arising out of the external and middle part of the Bone of the Elbow, and passing under the Annular Ligament, cleaves to the Lateral and outward part of the Bones of the Fore-Finger.

The Little-Finger hath two proper Muscles, viz. an Extensor and an Abductor.

The Extensor springs from the lower part of the Condylus of the Arm-Bone, and is fasten'd by a double Tendon in the second Articulation of the Little-Finger, and in the Tendon of the Extensor of all the others. {48}

The Abductor, call'd also Hypothenar, hath its beginning in the small Bone of the Wrist, which is situated over the others, and is terminated in the first Bone of the Little-Finger on the outside.

* * * * *

CHAP. XI.

Of the Muscles of the Thighs, Legs, and Feet.

What are the Motions of the Thighs?

The Thigh performs five kinds of Motions; for it is bent, extended, drawn within side and without, and turn'd round: All these Motions are produc'd by the means of fourteen Muscles, viz. three Flexors, three Extensors, three Adductors, three Abductors, and two Obturators for the Circular Motion.

The Flexors of the Thigh are the Psoas, Iliacus, and Pectineus.

The Psoas or Lumbaris is situated inwardly in the Abdomen, on the side of the Vertebra's. It proceeds from the transverse Apophyses of the two lower Vertebra's of the Back, and of the upper of the Loins, and lying on the inner Face of the Os Ilion, sticks to the lesser Trochanter or Rotator.

The Iliacus Internus hath its Origine in all the Lips of the inner Cavity of the Os Ilion, and being joyn'd by a Tendon to the Lumbaris, is inserted with it in the lesser Trochanter. {49}

The Pectineus takes its rise from the fore-part of the Os Pubis, and is united before to the Thigh-Bone a little below the lesser Trochanter.

The Extensors of the Thigh are the Glutius Major, Medius, and Minimus.

The Glutius Major springs forth out of the lateral part of the Os Sacrum, as also the hinder and outer part of the Os Ilion and Coccyx, and enters into the Thigh-Bone, four Fingers breadth below the great Trochanter or Rotator, being the thickest of all the Muscles of the Body.

The Glutius Medius, deducing its Original from the hinder and outward part of the Os Ilion, is inserted three Fingers breadth below the great Trochanter.

The Glutius Minimus ariseth from the bottom of the Cavity of the Os Ilion, and is fasten'd to a small Hole near the great Trochanter.

The Adductors of the Thigh are the Triceps Superior, Medius, and Inferior.

The Triceps Superior hath its beginning in the top of the Os Pubis, and is terminated in the top of a Line, which is on the inside of the Thigh.

The Triceps Medius proceeding from the middle of the Os Pubis, is inserted in the Thigh-Bone a little lower than the Triceps Superior.

The Triceps Inferior hath its Source in the bottom of the Os Pubis, and is implanted in the Thigh-Bone, a little lower than the Triceps Medius. Some Anatomists make only one Muscle of these three, attributing thereto three Originals and three Insertions. These Muscles serve to draw the Thighs one against another.

The Abductors of the Thigh are the Iliacus Externus, or Pyriformis, the Quadratus, and the Gemelli. {50}

The Pyriformis arising from the upper and lateral part of the Os Sacrum, and the the Os Ilion cleaves to the Neck of the great Trochanter.

The Quadratus or square Muscle of the Thigh takes its Origine from the external Prominence of the Os Ischion, and adheres to the outward part of the great Trochanter.

The Gemelli or Twin Muscles arise from two small Knobs in the hinder-part of the Ischion and insinuate themselves into a small Cavity in the Neck of the great Trochanter.

The Circular Motion of the Thigh is performed by the means of two Muscles, named the Obturatores Externi and Interni.

The Obturator Internus springs from the inner Circumference of the Oval Hole of the Ischion and its Tendons passing between the two Gemelli are inserted in a small Cavity at the Root of the great Trochanter or Rotator.

The Obturator Externus ariseth from the outward Circumference of the same Hole of one Ischion, and is terminated in the side of the other near the great Trochanter.

What are the Motions of the Leg, and what are its Muscles?

The Leg is mov'd four several ways, that is to say, it is bent, extended, and drawn inward and outward, by the means of eleven Muscles viz. three Flexors, four Extensors, two Adductors and two Abductors.

The three Flexors of the Leg are the Biceps, the Semi-nervosus, and the Semi-membranosus.

The Biceps hath two Heads, the longer whereof cometh out of the bottom of the Prominence {51} of the Ischion, and the other from the middle and exterior part of the Femur, and is terminated in the outward and upper part of the Epiphysis of the Perone or Fibula.

The Semi-nervosus hath its Origine in the Knob of the Ischion, and is join'd backward to the top of the Epiphysis of the Tibia. These three Muscles are plac'd in the back-part of the Thigh below the Buttocks.

The four Extensors of the Leg are the Rectus, the Vastus Internus, the Vastus Externus, and the Crureus.

The Rectus or streight Muscle of the Leg takes its rise from the fore-part and the bottom of the Ilion, and descends in a right Line: It covers with its Tendon, which is common to the three following, the whole Knee-Pan, and adheres to the top of the Tibia, on the fore-part.

The Vastus Internus, being situated on the inside of the Thigh, hath its beginning in the top of the Thigh inwardly, and a little below the lesser Trochanter or Rotator: Afterward it is ty'd to the Tibia by a large Tendon, common thereto with the preceeding.

The Vastus Externus is plac'd on the outside of the Thigh, springing from the top and the fore-part of the Femur, being united by the same Tendon with the two preceeding.

The Crureus proceeds from the top, and the fore-part of the Thigh-Bone, between the two Trochanters; then covering the whole Bone, it is also fasten'd to the Leg-Bone with the three preceeding Muscles, after having cover'd the Knee-Pan with their common {52} Tendon, which serves likewise as a Ligament to the Knee.

The two Adductors of the Leg are the Sartorius and the Gracilis.

The Sartorius or the Longissimus draws the leg inward, deriving its Original from the upper Spine of the Ischion; from whence it descends obliquely thro' the inside of the Thigh, and cleaves to the top on the inside of the Tibia.

The Gracilis hath its Origine in the fore-part at the bottom of the Os Pubis, and its Insertion in the top of the Tibia on the inside.

The two Abductors of the Leg are the Fascia lata, and the Poplitis.

The Fascia lata, or the Membranosus, is as it were a kind of large Band, which covers all the Muscles of the Thigh. It proceeds from the outward Lip of the Os Ilion, is ty'd by a large Membrane to the top of the Perone or Fibula and sometimes descends to the end of the Foot.

The Poplitis, or Sub-poplitis, arises from the lower and external Condylus of the Thigh-Bone, passeth obliquely from the outside to the inside, till it is lost in the upper and inner part of the Leg-Bone under the Ham.

What are the Motions of the Foot, and what are its Muscles?

The Foot performs two Motions by the help of nine Muscles, as being bent by two, and extended by seven.

The two Flexors are the Crureus Anticus, and the Peronius Anticus.

The Crureus or Tibius Anticus, is plac'd along the Tibia, and takes its rise from its upper and fore-part: Afterward it is bound by two {53} Tendons to the first Os Cuneiforme, or Wedge-like Bone, and to that of the Metatarsus or Instep, which stayeth the great Toe, after having pass'd under the annular Ligament.

The Peronius Anticus springs from the middle and outward-part of the Perone or Fibula, and insinuating it self thro' the Cleft which is under the external Malleolus before, sticks to the Bone of the Metatarsus that supports the little Toe.

The seven Extensors of the Foot are the two Gemelli, or the Soleus, the Plantaris, the Crureus Posticus, and the two Postici.

The Gemelli are the Interior and the Exterior; the former having its Source in the inner Condylus, and the other in the outward and lower of the Thigh-Bone; from whence they extend themselves till they are fasten'd to the Talus or Ankle-Bone by a Tendon common to them, with the two following.

The Soleus ariseth from the top on the back-part of the Leg-Bone and Perone, and confounding its Tendon with that of the Gemelli, sticks close to the Talus.

The Plantaris, which lies hid between the Gemelli and the Soleus, hath its Origine from the Exterior Condylus of the Thigh-Bone; then uniting its Tendon with the preceeding, it adheres to them; and this common Tendon is call'd Chorda Achillis.

The Crureus or Tibius Posticus, springs from the back-part of the Leg-Bone, from whence extending it self downward, it passeth thro' the Fissure in the Internal Malleolus, and cleaves to the inner-part of the Os Scaphoides. {54}

The Fibula Postici, are otherwise call'd the Longus and the Brevis, whereof one proceeds from the upper and almost fore-part of the Perone, terminating in the upper-part of the Bone, that supports the great Toe in the Metatarsus, and the other from the lower part of the Perone, adhering in like manner to the Bone with which the little Toe is sustain'd.

With what Motions are the Toes endu'd, how many Muscles have they, and which be they?

The Toes are bent and extended, as also drawn inward and outward, by the means of twenty two Muscles, of which sixteen are Common, and six Proper. The former are two Flexors, two Extensors, four Lumbricales, and eight Interossei. The first Flexor is nam'd Sublimis, and the other Profundus.

The Sublimis or Perforatus derives its Original from the lower and inner-part of the Talus and is fixt in its proper place by four cleft Tendons, which are inserted in the upper-part of the Bones of the first Phalanx of the four Toes. It is situated under the Sole of the Feet.

The Profundus or Perforans hath its beginning in the top and back-part of the Leg-Bone and Perone, slips under the Malleolus Internus thro' the Sinus Calcaris, and makes four Tendons which pass thro' the Fissures of the Tendon of the Sublimis, and cleaves to the Bones of the last Phalanx of the Toes, to bow them.

The first Extensor is call'd the Common, and the other the Pedias.

The Common Extensor, or the Longus, takes its rise from the top and fore-part of the Tibia in the place of its joyning with the Perone or {55} Fibula, and divides it self into four Tendons, which after having pass'd under the Annular Ligament, are inserted in the Articulations of every Toe.

The Pedias or the Brevis, being plac'd over the Foot, proceeds from the Annular Ligament, and the lower-part of the Perone, and sends forth four Tendons, which are fixt to the first Articulation of the four Toes on the outside, Thus this Muscle, together with the Longus, causeth their Extension.

The four Lumbrical Muscles of the Toes arise from the Tendons of the Profundus, and a Mass of Flesh at the Sole of the Feet. They are joyn'd by their Tendons with those of the Interossei Interni, and adhere inwardly to the side of the first Bones of the four Toes, to incline them toward the great Toe.

The Abductors, or those Muscles that remove the Toes from the great Toe, are the eight Interossei, whereof four are call'd Externi, and as many Interni. The former take their rise in the Spaces between the Bones of the Metatarsus, and are terminated outwardly in the side of the first Bones of the Toes. The Internal lie in the bottom of the Foot, and take up the Spaces between the five Bones of the Metatarsus. They arise from the Bones of the Tarsus, and the Intervals between those of the Metatarsus, and are implanted with the four Lumbricales inwardly, in the upper-part of the Bones of the first Phalanx of the four Toes.

Of the six Proper Muscles of the Toes, there are four appointed for the great Toe, which cause it to perform the Motions of Flexion, {56} Extension, and drawing forward or backward. The two others are the Adductor of the second Toe to the great Toe, and the Abductor of the little Toe, call'd Hypothenar.

The Proper Flexor of the great Toe, arises from the top of the Perone or Fibula, on the back part, passeth thro' the Ancle-Bone on the inside to the sole of the Foot, and is fasten'd to the Bone of the last Phalanx.

The Proper Extensor of the great Toe springs from the middle of the fore-part of the Perone, passeth over the Foot, and hath its Insertion in the upper-part of the Bone of the great Toe.

The Proper Adductor of the great Toe, or the Thenar, taking its rise inwardly on the side of the Talus, the Ossa Schaphoidea and Innominata, extends it self over the outward-part of the Bone of the Metatarsus, which stayeth the great Toe, and adheres to the top of the second Bone of the great Toe, which it draws inward.

The proper Abductor of the great Toe, or the Antithenar, draws it toward the other Toes. It derives its Origine from the Bone of the Metatarsus, which supports the little Toe, slides obliquely over the other Bones, and cleaves to the first Bone of the great Toe on the inside.

The Adductor appropriated to the second Toe hath its Source in the first Bone of the great Toe, on the inside, and sticks close to the Bones of the second Toe, which it draws to the great Toe. {57}

The Abductor of the little Toe, or the Hypothenar, proceeds from the outward part of the Bone of the Metatarsus, that stayeth the little Toe, and is inserted in the top of the little Toe, on the outside, to remove it from the others.

A List of all the Muscles in the Humane Body.

The Fore-head hath two Muscles 2 The hinder-part of the Head 2 The Eye-Lids 4 The Eyes 12 The Nose 7 The Ears on the outside 8 The Ears on the inside 6 The Lips 13 The Tongue 8 The Uvula, or Palate of the Mouth 4 The Larynx 13 The Pharynx 7 The Os Hyoides 10 The Lower Jaw 12 The Head 14 The Neck 8 The Omoplat?or Shoulder-Blades 8 The Arms 18 The Elbows 12 The Radii 8 The Wrists 12 The Fingers 48 The Breast, or the Parts of Respiration 57 The Loins 6 The Abdomen or lower Belly 10 The Testicles 2 The Bladder 1 {58} The Penis 4 The Clitoris 4 The Anus 3 The Thighs 30 The Legs 22 The Feet 18 The Toes 44 Total 425

* * * * *

CHAP. XII.

Of the Anatomy of the Nerves, Arteries, and Veins in general.

What is the Structure of the Nerves?

The Nerves are round white Bodies enclos'd in a double Membrane, communicated to them from the two Meninges of the Brain: Their Office is to convey the Animal Spirits into all the Parts.

Where is the Root and first beginning of all the Nerves?

All the Nerves take their Original from the Medulla Oblongata, and that of the Spine.

How is the distribution of them made thro' the whole Body?

It is directly perform'd by Conjugations or Pairs, whereof one goes to the Right-hand, and the other to the Left: There are nine Pairs of them that proceed from the Medulla Oblongata and enter into the Skull; and a Tenth that comes from the Marrow which lies between the Occipital and the first Vertebra of the Neck. It {59} passeth thro' the Hole of the Dura Mater, thro' which the Vertebral Artery enters, to distribute its Branches into several Parts.

To what Use are the nine Pairs of Nerves appropriated, which proceed from the Root of the Brain?

They are chiefly design'd for the Senses, and also for the Motion of their Organs, of which the Ancients discover'd only seven.

The first Pair of Nerves is call'd the Olfactory, and serves for the Smelling.

The second Pair is the Optici or Visorii Nervi, and bestows upon the Eyes the Faculty of seeing.

The third is term'd Motorii Oculorum, being serviceable for the Motion of the Eyes.

The fourth Pair is nam'd Oculorum Pathetici, which shews the Passion of the Mind in the Eyes, whereto it imparts a String as well as to the Lips.

The fifth is call'd the Gustative, and appropriated to the Taste, because it sends Twigs more especially to the Tongue, as also to the Fore-head, Temples, Face, Nostrils, Teeth, and Privy-Parts.

The Sixth is likewise for the Taste, and goes to the Palate.

The seventh is the Auditive Nerve, that enters into the Os Petrosum, where it divides it self into many Branches, which when gone forth, are distributed to the Muscles of the Tongue, Lips, Mouth, Face, Fore-head, Eye-Lids, &c.

The eighth is the Os Vagum, or wandering Pair, which is united to the Intercostal Nerve, as also to the Recurrent, Diaphragmatick, Mesenterick, &c. {60}

The ninth Pair, after having form'd a Trunk with the eighth, disperseth its Twigs several ways, whereof one is join'd with the Twig to the tenth, to be distributed together into the Muscle Sternohyoideus, and into the Tongue.

The Intercostal and Spinal are not Pairs of Nerves, but only Branches or Twigs of other Pairs.

What is the Distribution and Use of the thirty Pairs of Nerves that proceed from the Spinal Marrow?

There are seven that go forth from the several Vertebra's of the Neck, twelve from those of the Back, five from the Loins, and six from the Os Sacrum, according to the following Progression.

The first of the seven Pairs of Nerves of the Neck proceeds from between the Occipital Bone and the first Vertebra, nam'd Atlas, its Fibres being lost in the Muscles of the hinder-part of the Head and Neck.

The second Pair springs from between the first and second Vertebra of the Neck; the Fibres whereof are lost in the Muscles of the Head, and in the Skin of the Face.

The third Pair issueth from between the second and third Vertebra of the Neck; and its Fibres are lost in the Flexor Muscles and Extensors of the Neck.

The fourth, fifth, sixth, and seventh Pairs proceed from between the Vertebra's, as before, but their Fibres are lost in the Neck of the Omoplata, in the Arm, and in the Diaphragme or Midriff. Here it ought to be observ'd by the way that the Arms receive Branches not only from the {61} four last Pairs of the Nerves of the Neck, but also from the two first Pairs of the Back, which are extended even to the end of the Fingers: Whence it happens that in the Palsie of the Arms, Remedies are usually apply'd to the Vertebra's of the Neck; and that in Phlebotomy or letting Blood, care must be taken to avoid pricking the Nerve, which accompanies the Basilick Vein in the Elbow.

The twelve Pairs of Nerves that have their Beginning from between the Vertebra's of the Back, are each of them divided into two Branches, as the others; and their Branches are distributed in like manner to the Muscles of the Breast, and to those of the Back and Abdomen.

The five Pairs which take their Rise from between the Vertebra's of the Loins, have thicker Branches than the others, and the distribution of them is made to the Muscles of the Loins, Hypogastrium, and Thighs.

Of the six Pairs of Nerves that proceed from the Os Sacrum, the four Upper with the three Lower of the Loins, send forth Fibres of Nerves to the Thigh, Leg, and Foot; and the two last Pairs impart Nerves to the Anus, Bladder, and privy Parts.

What is the Structure of the Arteries?

The Arteries are long and round Canals, consisting of four sorts of Tunicks or Membranes, which have their Rise from the left Ventricle of the Heart, from whence they receive the Blood, and convey it to all the Parts of the Body for their Nourishment.

What is the Construction of these four Tunicks or Membranes of the Arteries? {62}

The first being thin and Nervous in its outward Superficies, is in the Inside a Plexus or Interlacement of small Veins and Arteries, and Fibres of Nerves, which enter into the other following Tunicks, to nourish them.

The second sticking close to the former, is altogether full of whitish Glandules, that serve to separate the serous Particles of the Blood.

The third is intirely Musculous, and interwoven with Annular Fibres.

The fourth is very thin, and hath its Fibres all streight.

Whence proceeds the Pulse or beating of the Arteries?

It is deriv'd from the Heart, and exactly answers to its Motion of Diastole and Systole.

By what Name is the first Trunk of the Arteries call'd, and what is the Effect of the Distribution made thence to the whole Body?

The first Trunk of the Arteries is nam'd Aorta, or the thick Artery, which proceeds immediately from the left Ventricle of the Heart, whereto it communicates before its departure from the Pericardium, one or two small Branches call'd the Coronary: Afterward it is divided into two Branches, whereof one goes upward, and is term'd the Ascending Artery; and the other downward, under the Denomination of the Descending Artery.

The Ascending Artery ariseth upward along the Aspera Arteria or Wind-Pipe, to the Clavicles, and is there divided into two Branches, call'd the Subclavian Arteries, one whereof goes forward to the Right side, and the other to the Left; and they both send forth on each side {63} divers Branches, which take their Names from the several Parts, whereto they are distributed; such are the Carotides or Soporales Interni & Externi, which pass to the Head; the Mediastina; the Intercostal; the Axillar, and others.

The Descending Artery, before its departure from the Breast, affords certain Branches to the Pericardium, Diaphragm, and lower Ribs; afterward it penetrates the Diaphragm, and constitutes seven double Branches. The first is of those that are call'd Coeliack, and which go to the Liver and Spleen. The second Branch contains the Upper Mesenterick. The third the Emulgent, which pass to the Reins. The fourth the Spermatick, which are extended to the Genitals. The fifth the Lower Mesenterick. The sixth the Lumbar. And the seventh the Muscular. But assoon as the great Trunk is come downward to the Os Sacrum, it divides it self into two thick Arteries nam'd the Iliack, which are distributed on both sides, each of them making two Internal and External Branches, which likewise impart Sprigs or lesser Arteries, to the Bladder, Anus, Matrix, and other adjacent Parts: Then the Master-Branch forms the Crural Arteries on the inside of the Thighs, which are communicated by multiplying their Number even to the ends of the Toes, in passing over the External Ancle-Bones of the Feet.

What is the Structure of the Veins?

The Veins are long and round Canals made of four kinds of Tunicks or Membranes, whose Office it is to receive the Blood that remains after the Nourishment is taken, and to carry it back to the Heart to be reviv'd. {64}

What is the Form of the four Tunicks that make the Canals of the Veins?

The first is a Contexture of Nervous and streight Fibres. The second is a Plexus of small Vessels that carry the Nourishment. The third is all over beset with Glandules thro' which are filtrated the serous Particles of the Blood contain'd in the Vessels of the second Tunicle. The fourth is a Series of Annular and Musculous or Fleshy Fibres.

Which are the most numerous, the Arteries or the Veins?

The Number of the Veins exceeds that of the Arteries; and there are scarce any Arteries without Veins accompanying them.

Where is the Beginning and Original of all the Veins?

All the Veins have their Root in the Liver, and two of the three great Trunks that proceed from thence, are call'd Vena Port? and Vena Cava; and the third is twofold, viz. the ascending and the descending.

The Vena Port?is distributed to all the Parts contain'd in the lower Belly, and terminated in the Fundament; where it makes the Internal Hemorrhoidal Veins.

The Vena Cava is immediately divided into two thick Branches, one whereof ariseth upward to the Right Ventricle of the Heart, and forms the ascending Vena Cava; as the other goes downward to the Feet, and constitutes the descending.

What is the Distribution of the ascending Vena Cava?

It perforates the Diaphragm, goes to the Heart, and ascends from thence to the Clavicles, {65} after having communicated to the Midriff in passing, a small Branch call'd the Phrenicus; as also one or two to the Heart, nam'd the Coronary; and some others to the upper Ribs, besides the single Branch, term'd Azygos, only on the right side. But the Trunk of the ascending Vena Cava, being once come up to the Clavicles, is divided into two Branches, well known by the Name of the Subclavian, one whereof Shoots forth toward the Right side, and the other toward the Left; and they both make various Ramifications like to those of the thick ascending Artery, by producing the Cervicalis or Soporalis, and the Internal and External Jugulars that go to the Head; as also the Axillars, which pass to the Arms and Shoulders, forming the Cephalick, the Median, and the Basilick on the inside of the Elbow.

The descending Vena Cava in like manner accompanieth the Ramifications of the Aorta, or thick descending Artery, to the fourth Vertebra of the Loins, where it sends forth two Branches, nam'd the Iliack, one whereof goes to the Right side, and the other to the Left, both inwardly and outwardly; imparting divers Twigs or lesser Branches to all the Parts contain'd in the Abdomen or lower Belly, even as far as the Fundament, where it makes the External Hemorrhoidal Veins. Afterward the outward Branch of the Iliack descends in the Thigh, to form the Crural, and others, as far as the Saphea, together with those that are situated at the end of the Feet.

* * * * *

{66}

CHAP XII.

Of the Anatomy of the Abdomen, or lower Belly.

What is the clearest Division of the Human Body into various Parts, and that which is most followed in the Anatomical Schools?

It is that which constitutes three Venters, that is to say, the Upper, the Middle, and the Lower, which are the Head, the Thorax or Breast and the Abdomen or lower Belly, together with the Extremities, which are the Arms and Legs.

What is the lower Belly?

It is a Cavity of the Body that contains the nourishing parts, as the Reins, the Bladder, and all those that are appropriated to Generation in both Sexes.

What is to be consider'd outwardly in the lower Belly?

Its different Regions, and the several parts therein contain'd.

What are these Regions?

They are the Epigastrick, the Umbilical, and the Hypogastrick.

What is their Extent?

It is from the Xyphoides or Sword-like Cartilage to the Os Pubis, the division whereof into three equal Parts, constitutes the three different Regions; the Epigastrium being the first upward, the Umbilicus the second, and the Hypogastrium the third. {67}

What Are the Parts contain'd in the Epigastrium, and what Place do they possess therein?

The Parts contain'd in the Epigastrium are the Liver, the Spleen, the Stomach, and the Pancreas or Sweet-bread, which lies underneath: The Stomach takes up the middle before, the Liver being plac'd on the Right side, and the Spleen on the Left; so that these two sides of the Epigastrick Region, are call'd the Right and Left Hypochondria.

What Parts are there contain'd in the Umbilical Region, and what is their situation?

They are the most part of the thin Intestines or small Guts, viz. the Duodenum, the Jejunum, and the Ileon, which have their Residence in the middle, where they are encircled with a Portion of the two great Guts, Cecum and Colon, that take possession of the Sides, otherwise call'd the Flanks. The Reins or Kidneys are also in this Place, above, and somewhat backward.

What Parts are there contain'd in the Hypogastrium, and of what Place are they possest?

The greater part of the thick-Guts, Coecum, and Colon, are enclos'd therein, with the entire Rectum; there is also a Portion of the Ileon, which hides it self in the sides of the Ilia, or Hip-Bones: In the middle under the Os Pubis, the Bladder is situated on the Gut Rectum in Men, and the Matrix in Women lies between the Rectum and Bladder.

After what manner is the opening of a Corps or dead Body perform'd at a publick Dissection? {68}

It is begun with a Crucial Incision in the Skin from underneath the Throat downward, traversing from one side to another in the Umbilical Region; then this Skin is pull'd off at the four Corners, and the Panicula Adiposa is immediately discover'd: Under this Fat lies a Fleshy Membrane, call'd Membrana Carnosa; and after that, the common Membrane of all the Muscles of the lower Belly. Thus we have taken a View of what Anatomists commonly term the five Teguments, that is to say, the Epiderma or Scarf-Skin, the Derma or true Skin, the Panicula Adiposa, the Panicula Carnosa or Membranus Carnosa, and the common Membrane of the Muscles.

The five Teguments being remov'd, we meet with as many Muscles on each side, viz. the descending Oblique, the ascending Oblique, the Transverse, the streight, and the Pyramidal, by the means whereof the Belly is extended and contracted. Afterwards appears a Membrane nam'd Peritoneum, which contains all the Bowels, and covers the whole lower Belly, being strongly fasten'd to the first and third Vertebra's of the Back. The Fat skinny Net which lies immediately under the Peritoneum, is call'd Epiploon and Omentum, or the Caul; it floats over the Bowels, keeping them in a continual Suppleness necessary for their Functions, maintains the Heat of the Stomach, and contributes to Digestion.

It remains to take an Account of the Bowels viz. the Stomach, Mesentery, Liver, Spleen, Kidneys, Bladder, and Guts, together with the Parts appointed for Generation, which in Men {69} are the Spermatick Vessels, the Testicles, and the Penis; and in Women, the Spermatick Vessels, the Testicles or Ovaries, the Matrix, and its Vagina or Neck.

What is the Stomach?

It is the Receptacle of the Aliments or Food convey'd thither thro' the Oesophagus or Gullet, which is a Canal, or kind of streight Gut that reacheth from the Throat to the Mouth of the Stomach. The Stomach it self is situated immediately under the Diaphragm or Midriff, between the Liver and the Spleen, having two Orifices, whereof the Left is properly call'd Stomachus, or the Upper, and the Right (at its other Extremity) Pylorus, or the lower Orifice. Its Figure resembleth that of a Bag-Pipe, and the greater part of its Body lies toward the Left side. It is compos'd of three Membranes, viz. one Common, which it receives from the   Peritoneum; and two Proper; the two uppermost being smooth, and the innermost altogether wrinkled.

What is the Pancreas or Sweet-bread?

It is a Fat Body, consisting of many Glandules wrapt up in the same Tunicle, being situated under the Pylorus or lower Orifice of the Stomach: It helps Digestion, and hath divers other uses; but its principal Office is to separate the serous Particles of the Blood, to be convey'd afterward into the Gut Duodenum, by a Canal or Passage, nam'd the Pancreatick. This Juice serves to cause the Chyle to ferment with the Choler, in order to remove the grosser Particles from those that ought to enter into the Lacteal Vessels.

Into how many sorts are the Guts distinguish'd? {70}

There are two sorts, viz. the thin and the thick.

How many thin or small Guts are there?

Three; that is to say, the Duodenum, the Jejunum, and the Ileon.

How many thick Guts are there?

Three likewise; viz. the Coecum, the Colon, and the Rectum.

Why are some of them call'd thin Guts, and others thick?

Because the thin are smaller, being appointed only to transport the Chyle out of the Stomach into the Reserver; whereas the thick are more large and stronger, serving to carry forth the gross Excrements out of the Belly.

Are the six Guts of an equal length?

No, the Duodenum, which is the first of the thin Guts, is only twelve Fingers breadth long. The Jejunum, being the second, so call'd because always empty, is five Foot long: The third is nam'd Ileon, by reason of its great Turnings which oblige it to pass to the Os Ilion, where it produceth a Rupture; it extends it self almost twenty Foot in length.

The first of the thick Guts, known by the Name of Coecum, is very short, and properly only an Appendix or Bag of a Finger's length. That which follows is the Colon, being the largest of all, and full of little Cells, which are fill'd sometimes with Wind and other Matters that excite the Pains of the Colick. It encompasseth the thin Guts, in passing from the top to the bottom of the Belly, by the means of its great Circumvolutions, and is from eight to nine Foot long. The last is the Rectum or {71} streight Gut, so nam'd, because it goes directly to the Fundament: It is no longer than ones Hand, but it is fleshy, and situated upon the Os Sacrum, and the Coccyx or Rump-Bone.

What is the Peristaltick Motion of the Guts?

It is the successive Motion and Undulation, whereby the Guts insensibly push forward from the top to the bottom, the Matters contain'd in them; and that Motion which on the contrary is perform'd from the bottom to the top, is term'd the Antiperistaltick as it happens in the Iliack Passion, or twisting of the Guts, call'd Domine Miserere, by reason of its intolerable Pain.

What is the Mesentery?

It is a kind of Membrane somewhat fleshy, which is join'd to the Spine in the bottom and middle of the Belly, and by its folding, keeps all the Guts steady in their place; it is all over beset with red, white, and Lymphatick Vessels; that is to say, those that carry the Blood, Chyle, and Lympha, which serves to cause this last to run more freely, and to ferment. Three notable Glandules are also observ'd therein, the greatest whereof lies in the middle, and is nam'd Asellius's Pancreas; the two other lesser are call'd Lumbar Glandules, as being situated near the Left Kidney. From each of these Glandules proceeds a small Branch; and both are united together to make the great Lacteal Vein, or Thoracick Canal. This Tube conveys the Chyle along the Vertebra's of the Back to the Left Subclavian Vein; from whence it passeth into the ascending Vena Cava, and descends in the Right Ventricle of the Heart, {72} where it assumes the form of Blood; from whence it passeth to the Lungs thro' the Pulmonary Artery; then it returns to the Heart thro' the Pulmonary Vein, and goes forth again thro' the Left Ventricle of the Heart, between the Aorta or great Artery, to be afterward distributed to all the Parts of the Body. This is the ordinary Passage for the Circulation of the Chyle, and the Sanguification of the Heart.

What is the Liver?

The Liver, being the thickest of all the Bowels, is plac'd in the Right Hypochondrium, at the distance only of a Fingers breadth from the Diaphragm; its Figure much resembling that of a thick piece of Beef: It is Convex on the outside, and Concave within; its Substance is soft and tender, its Colour and Consistence being like coagulated Blood: It is cleft at bottom, and divided into two Lobes, viz. one greater, and the other less: Its Office is to purifie the Mass of Blood by Filtration; and it is bound by two strong Ligaments, the first whereof adheres to the Diaphragm, and the second to the Xiphoides or Sword-like Cartilage. Two great Veins take their Rise from hence, viz. the Vena Port? and the Vena Cava, which form innumerable Branches, as it were Roots in the Body of the Liver. The Gall-Bladder is fasten'd to the hollow part thereof, and dischargeth its Choler into the Gut Duodenum, thro' the Vessels that bear the Name of Meatus Choledochi, or Ductus Biliares. This Choler is not a meer Excrement, but on the contrary of singular Use in causing the Fermentation of the Chyle, and bringing it to perfection. {73}

What is the Spleen?

The Spleen is a Bowel resembling a Hart's Tongue in shape, and situated in the Left Hypochondrium, over-against the Liver: Its length is about half a Foot, and its breadth equal to that of three Fingers; its Substance being soft, as that of the Liver, and its Colour like dark coagulated Blood: It is fasten'd to the Peritoneum, Left Kidney, Diaphragm, and to the Caul on the inside; as also to the Stomach by certain Veins, call'd Vasa Brevia; nevertheless these Ligatures do not hinder it from wandering here and there in the lower Belly, where it often changeth its place, and causeth many dreadful symptoms by its irregular Motions. Its Office is to Subtilize the Blood by cleansing and refining it.

What are the Reins?

The Reins or Kidneys are Parts of a Fleshy Consistence, harder and more firm than that of the Liver and Spleen: They are both situated in the sides of the Umbilical Region, upon the Muscle Psoas, between the two Tunicks of the Peritoneum; but the Right is lower than the Left: Their Shape resembleth that of a French Bean, and they receive Nerves from the Stomach, whence Vomitings are frequently occasion'd in the Nephritical Colicks: They are fasten'd to the Midriff, Loins, and Aorta, by the Emulgent Arteries; as also to the Bladder by the Ureters. The Right Kidney likewise adheres to the Gut Cecum, and the Left to the Colon. Their Office is to filtrate or strain the Urine in the Pelves or Basons, which they have in the middle of their Body on the inside, and {74} to cause it to run thro' the Vessels call'd Ureters into the Bladder.

Immediately above the Reins on each side, is a flat and soft Glandule, of the thickness of a Nut; they are nam'd Renal Glandules, or Capsul?Atribiliari? because they contain a blackish Liquor, which (as they say) serves as it were Leaven for the Blood, to set it a fermenting.

What is the Bladder?

It is the Bason or Reserver of Urines, of a Membranous Substance as the Stomach, being plac'd in the middle of the Hypogastrick Region; so that it is guarded by the Os Sacrum behind, and by the Os Pubis before: Two Parts are to be distinguish'd therein, viz. its Bottom and Top; by its Membranous Bottom it is join'd to the Navel, and suspended by the means of the Urachus, and the two Umbilical Arteries which degenerate into Ligaments in adult Persons: As by its fleshy Neck, longer and crooked in Men, and shorter and streight in Women it cleaves to the Intestinum Rectum in the former, and to the Neck of the Womb in the latter. Lastly, its Office is to receive the Urines to keep them, and to discharge them from time to time.

What are the Genitals in Men?

They are the Spermatick Vessels, the Testicles, and the Penis. The Spermatick Vessels are a Vein and an Artery on each side; the former proceeding from the Aorta, or thick Artery of the Heart; and the other from the Branches of the Vena Cava of the Liver. These Arteries and Veins are terminated in the Body of the {75} Testicles, which are two in Number, enclos'd within the Scrotum.

The Office of the Testicles is to filtrate the Seed, which is brought thither from all the parts of the Body, thro' the Spermatick Vessels, called Pr 鍣 arantia, and afterwards to cause it to pass thro' others nam'd Deferentia, to the Vesicul?Seminales, from whence it is forc'd into the Ureter, thro' two small and very short Canals.

The Penis or Yard is a Nervous and Membranous Part, well furnish'd with Veins and Arteries, containing in the middle the Canal of the Ureter: Its Extremity, which consists of a very delicate and spongy sort of Flesh, is call'd Balanus, or Glans, and the Nut, the Skin that covers it being nam'd the Prutrium, or the Fore-Skin. Thus by the means of this swell'd Part, and stiff thro' the affluence of the Spirits, the Male injects his Seed into the Matrix of the Female, to propagate his Kind.

What are the Parts appropriated to Generation in Women?

They are the Spermatick Vessels, the Ovaries or Testicles, and the Matrix. The Spermatick Vessels are a Vein and an Artery on each side, as in Men: The Ovaries or Testicles, situated on the side of the bottom of the Matrix, are almost of the same bigness with those of Men, but of a round and flat Figure. The Vesicul? or little Bladders which they contain, are usually term'd Ova or

Eggs by Modern Anatomists; and the Vessels that pass from these Testicles or Ovaries to the Cornua of the Uterus, are call'd Deferentia or Ejaculatoria. {76}

The Matrix, Uterus or Womb, is the principal Organ of Generation, and the place where it is perform'd, resembling the Figure of a Pear with its Head upward, and being situated between the Gut Rectum and the Bladder: It is of a fleshy and membranous Substance, retain'd in its place by four Ligaments, fasten'd to the bottom; whereof the two upper are large ones, proceeding from the Loins, and the two lower round, taking their Rise from the Groin, where they form a kind of Goose-Foot, which is extended to the Os Pubis, and the flat part of the Thighs; which is the cause that Women are in danger of Miscarrying when they fall upon their Knees.

The Exterior Neck of the Womb, call'd Vagina, is made almost in form of a Throat or Gullet, extending it self outwardly to the sides of the Lips of the Pudendum, and being terminated inwardly at the internal Orifice of the Matrix, the shape whereof resembleth that of the Muzzle or Nose of a little Dog. The outward Neck of the womb is fasten'd to the Bladder and the Os Pubis before, and in the hinder part to the Os Sacrum: Between the Lips of the Pudendum lie the Nymph? which are plac'd at the Extremity of the Canal of the Bladder, to convey the Urines; and somewhat farther appear four Caruncles, or small pieces of Flesh, at the Entrance of the Vagina, which when join'd together make the thin Membrane call'd Hymen.

* * * * *

{77}

CHAP. XIV.

Of the Anatomy of the Thorax, Breast, or middle Venter.

What is the Breast?

It is a Cavity in which the Heart and the Lungs are principally enclos'd.

What is to be consider'd outwardly in the Breast?

Its extent, and the situation of the Parts therein contain'd.

What is its extent?

It is extended from the Clavicles to the Xiphoides, or Sword-like Cartilage on the fore-part, and bounded on the hinder by the twelfth Vertebra of the Back, having all the Ribs to form its Circumference, and the Diaphragm for its Bounds at bottom, separating it from the Abdomen or lower Belly.

What is the situation of the Parts contain'd in the Breast?

The Lungs take up the upper Region, and fill almost the whole Space, descending at the distance of two Fingers breadth from the Diaphragm; the Heart is situated in the middle, bearing its Point somewhat towards the Left side, under the Lobes of the Lungs, which are divided by the Mediastinum that distinguishes them into the Right and Left Parts.

How is the Breast Anatomiz'd or open'd? {78}

After the dissection of the five Teguments, and the removal of the Muscles, as in the lower Belly, the Anatomist proceeds to lift up the Sternum or Breast-Bone, by separating it from the Ribs; then it is laid upon the Face, or else entirely taken away, to the end that the internal Parts of the Breast may be more clearly discover'd; whereupon immediately appear, the Heart, the Lungs, the Diaphragm, and the Mediastinum, which sticks to the Sternum throughout its whole length.

What is the Heart?

It is a most noble Part, being the Fountain of Life, and the first Original of the Motion of all the others; on which account it is call'd Primus vivens, & ultimum moriens; that is to say, the first Member that begins to live, and the last that dies.

What Parts are to be consider'd in the Heart?

Its fleshy Substance, with all its Fibres turn'd round like the Skrews of a Vice; its Basis, Point, Auricles, Ventricles, large Vessels, Pericardium and Ligatures or Tyes: The Basis is the uppermost and broadest part; the Point is the lowermost and narrowest part; the two Auricles or small Ears being as it were little Cisterns or Reservers, that pour the Blood by degrees into the Heart, are situated on each side above the Ventricles. The Ventricles, which are likewise two in Number, are certain Cavities in its Right and Left Sides. The large Vessels are the Aorta or great Artery, and the Vena Cava together with the Pulmonary Artery and Vein. The Pericardium is a kind of Bag fill'd with Water, wherein the Heart is kept; which is {79} fasten'd to the Mediastinum by its Basis, and to the large Vessels that enter and go out of its Ventricles.

What are the Terms appropriated to the continual beating of the Heart?

They are Diastole and Systole, from whence proceed two several Motions, the first whereof is that of Dilatation, and the other of Contraction, communicated to all the Arteries which have the same Pulse.

To what use serves the Water contain'd in the Pericardium?

It prevents the drying of the Heart by its perpetual Motion.

What are the Lungs?

They are an Organ serving for Respiration, of a soft Substance, and porous as a Sponge, being all over beset with Arteries, Veins, Nerves, and Lymphatick Vessels, and perforated with small Cartilaginous Tubes, that are imparted to it from the Wind-Pipe, and are call'd Bronchia. Their Natural Colour is a pale Red, and marbl'd dark Brown; and their whole Body is wrapt up in a fine smooth Membrane, which they receive from the Pleuron. They are suspended by the Wind-Pipe, by their proper Artery and Vein, and by the Ligatures that fasten them to the Sternum, Mediastinum, and frequently to the Pleuron it self: They are also divided into the Right and Left Parts by the Mediastinum; having four or five Lobes, whereof those on the Left side cover the Heart. Their continual Motion consists in Inspiration, to take in the Air, and Expiration, to drive it out. The Larynx makes the Entrance of the Wind-Pipe {80} into the Lungs, and the Pharynx that of the Oesophagus or Gullet, at the bottom of the Mouth to pass into the Stomach.

* * * * *

CHAP. XV.

Of the Anatomy of the Head, or upper Venter.

What is the head?

It is a bony Part, that contains and encloseth the Brain within its Cavity.

What is most remarkable in the outward parts of the Head?

The Temporal Arteries, the Crotaphit? or Temporal Muscles, and the Sutures of the Skull.

Why are these things considerable?

The Temporal Arteries are of good Note, because they are expos'd on the outside, lying even with the Skin. The Crotophite Muscles are so likewise, in regard that they cannot be hurt without danger of Convulsions, by reason of the Pericranium with which they are cover'd. And the Sutures, because the Meninges of the Brain proceed from thence to form the Pericranium.

What is the Pericranium?

It is a Membrane that lies under the thick hairy Skin of the Head, and immediately covers the Skull.

What are the Meninges?

They are two Membranes that enclose the Substance or Marrow of the Brain.

What is a Suture? {81}

It is a kind of thick Seam or Stitch, that serves to unite the Bones of the Skull.

How many sorts of Sutures are there?

There are two sorts, viz. the true, and the false or Bastard.

What are the true Sutures?

They are three in number, namely the Sagittal, the Coronal, and the Lambdoidal.

What is the disposition or situation of the true Sutures?

The Sagittal is streight, beginning in the middle of the Fore-head, and sometimes at the root of the Nose, and being terminated behind, at the joining of the two Branches of the Lambdoidal Suture.

The Coronal appears in form of a Crown, passing to the middle of the Head, and descending thro' the Temples, to finish its Circumference in the Root of the Nose.

The Lambdoidal Suture is made like an open Pair of Compasses, the Legs whereof are extended toward the Shoulders; and the Button is in the top of the Head backward.

What are the Bastard Sutures?

They are those that are call'd Squamous or scaly.

What is the disposition of natural situation of these false Sutures?

They are plac'd at the two sides of the Head, and make a Semi-Circle of the bigness of the Ears, round the same Ears.

What difference is there between the true and spurious Sutures.

The true Sutures are made in form of the Teeth of a Saw, which enter one into the other; and the false or Bastard ones are those that resemble the Scales of Fishes, which {82} are join'd together by passing one over the other.

What is the Use of the Sutures?

The Ancients were of Opinion, that they were made to hinder the Fracture of one Skull-Bone from passing thro' the whole Head; but there is more reason to believe that they have the three following Uses, that is to say, 1. To promote the transpiration of the Brain. 2. To give Passage to the Vessels that go to the Diploe. 3. To retain the Meninges, and to support the Mass of the Brain, which is cover'd by them.

What are the Names of the Bones that compose the Skull?

The Bone of the fore-part of the Head is call'd Sinciput, or the Fore-head-Bone, as also the Frontal or Coronal Bone. The Bone of the hinder-part, enclos'd within the Lambdoidal Suture, is term'd the Occipital. The two Bones that form the upper-part, and are distinguish'd by the Sagittal Suture, bear the Name of Parietals, one being on the Right side, and the other on the Left. And those behind the Ears are call'd Temporal, Squamosa, or Petrosa. These also are distinguish'd into the Right and Left Temporals, and are join'd to the bottom of the Parietal by a bastard squamous Suture.

What is most remarkable in the thickness of the Skull-Bones?

The Diploe, which is nothing else but a Plexus or Contexture of small Vessels, that nourish the Bones, and in the middle of their thickness make the distinction of the first and second Tablature of the Bones; whence it sometimes {83} happens that an exfoliative Trepan, or Semi-Trepan, is sufficient, when the first of these two Tables is only broken, the other remaining entire.

Is the Brain which is preserv'd in the Skull all of one Piece, or one equal Mass?

No, it is distinguish'd by the means of the Meninges into the Brain it self, and the Cerebellum or little Brain; the Brain, properly so called, takes up almost the whole Cavity of the Skull, and the Cerebellum is lodg'd altogether in the hinder-part, where it constitutes only one entire Body; whereas the former is divided into the Right and Left Parts by the Meninges, which cut it even to the bottom; whence these Foldings are call'd Falx; i. e. a Scythe or Sickle.

What is chiefly remarkable in the Substance of the Brain?

The Ventricles or Cavities which are found therein, together with the great Number of Veins, Arteries, Lymphatic Vessels, and Nerves, that carry Sense to all the Parts of the Body, and Spirits for their Motion.

An exact Historical Account of all the Holes of the Skull, and the Vessels that pass thro' them.

To attain to an exact Knowledge of all the Holes with which the inside of the Basis of the Skull is perforated, they are to be consider'd either with respect to the Nerves, or to the Sanguinary Vessels. {84}

There are nine Pairs of Nerves that arise from the Medulla Oblongata, and go forth out of the Skull through many Holes hereafter nam'd.

The first Pair is that of the Olfactory Nerves, appropriated to the Sense of Smelling, which are divided below the Os Cribiforme, or Sieve-like Bone, into divers Threads, that passing into the Nose through many Holes with which this Bone is pierc'd, are distributed to the inner Tunick of the Nose.

The second Pair is that of the Optick or Visual Nerves, that pass into the Orbits of the Eyes, thro' certain peculiar Holes made in the Os Sphenoides, or Wedge-like Bone, immediately above the Anterior Apophysis Clinoides.

In the Portion of the Os Sphenoides, that makes the Basis of the Orbit, lies a Fissure about seven or eight Hairs breadth long, which is to be observ'd chiefly at the bottom, that is to say, below the Hole, thro' which the Optick Nerve passeth; where it is almost round, and larger than at the top, where it is terminated in a very long and acute Angle.

There are many Pairs of Nerves that enter into the Orbit thro' this Fissure, viz. 1. The third Pair, call'd the Motorii Oculorum. 2. The fourth Pair, nam'd Pathetici, by Dr. Willis. And 3. The whole sixth Pair. Besides these three Pairs, which go entire thro' this Cleft, there is also a Passage for the upper Branch of the foremost Fibre of the fifth Pair, which the same renowned Physician calls the Ophthalmick Branch. Beyond the lower-part of the said Fissure, toward the hinder-part of the Head, is to be seen {85} in the Os Sphenoides on each side, a Hole that doth not penetrate the Basis of the Skull, but makes a kind of

Ductus, about an Hair's breadth long, which is open'd behind the Orbit on the top of the Space between the Apophysis Pterygoides, and the third Bone of the Jaw; thro' this Ductus runs the lower Branch of the foremost Fibre of the fifth Pair.

About the length of two Hairs breadth beyond these Ductus's, we may also discover in the Os Sphenoides, or Wedge-like Bone, two Holes of an Oblong and almost Oval Figure, which are plac'd in the hindermost sides of that of the Os Sphenoides, and gives passage to the hindermost Fibre of the fifth Pair.

The Hole thro' which runs the Auditory Nerve, that makes the seventh Pair, is in the middle of the hinder-part of the Os Petrosum, that looks toward the Cerebellum: This Hole being very large, is the Entrance of a Ductus that is hollow'd in the Os Petrosum, and which sinking obliquely from the fore-part backward, for the depth of about two Hairs breadth, forms as it were the bottom of a Sack, the lowermost part whereof is terminated partly by the Basis of the Cochlea, and partly by a Portion of the Mouth of the Vestibulum. At the bottom of this Ductus are many Holes, but the most considerable is that of the upper-part, thro' which passeth a Portion of the Auditory Nerve. This is also the Entrance of another Ductus made in the Os Petrosum, which is open'd between the Apophysis Mastoides and Styloides: These other Holes afford a Passage to the Branches of the soft Portion of the same Auditory Nerve. {86}

Below this Ductus there is a remarkable Hole form'd by the meeting of two hollow Cuts the larger whereof is in the Occipital Bone and the other in the lower-part of the Apophysis Petrosi: From the middle of the upper-part of this Hole issueth forth a small Prominence or bony Point, whereto is join'd an Appendix of the Dura Mater, which divides the Hole into two parts; so that thro' the foremost Orifice passeth the Nerve of the eighth Pair, and that which is call'd the Spinal Nerve. We shall have occasion hereafter to shew the Use of the hinder Orifice.

Near the great Hole of the Occipital Bone from whence proceeds the Medulla Oblongata, we may observe a Hole almost round and oblong thro' which passeth the Nerve of the ninth Pair. This Hole is entirely situated in the Occipital Bone, and making a little Way in the Bone passeth obliquely from the back-part forward. In the inside of the Skull this Hole is sometimes double, but its two Entrances are re-united in the outward-part of the Skull; and the two Branches that form the Origine of this Nerve and which pass thro' these two Holes, are likewise re-united at their Departure, These are the Passages of the nine Pairs of Nerves that proceed from the Medulla Oblongata, and it remains only to show that Paths thro' which the Intercostal Nerve goes forth, as also that of the tenth Pair. The Intercostal runs out of the Skull thro' the Ductus that gives Entrance to the Internal Carotick Artery. As for the tenth Pair, in regard that it ariseth from the Marrow which is enclos'd between the Occipital {87} Bone and the first Vertebra, it goes forth thro' the Hole of the Dura Mater, where the Vertebral Artery enters.

To know well the Holes thro' which the Vessels that belong to the inner-part of the Head enter, and issue forth, it is requisite to distinguish them into those which are distributed to the Dura Mater, and those that are appointed for the Brain. The Vessels of the Dura Mater, are Branches of the Carotick or Vertebral Arteries.

In the Os Sphenoides, or Wedge-like Bone, behind the Hole thro' which passeth the hindermost Fibre of the fifth Pair of Nerves lies another small Hole, almost round, that gives Entrance to a Branch of the External Carotick Artery, which in entring, immediately adheres to the Dura Mater, and forms many Ramifications to overspread the whole Portion of this Membrane, which covers the sides, and the upper-part of the Brain.

At the bottom and top of the lateral outward part of the Orbit of the Eye, above the acute Angle, for want of the Os Sphenoides, there is a Hole thro' which passeth an Artery, being a Twig of a Branch of the Internal Carotick, which is diffus'd in the Eye, and distributed to almost the whole Portion of the Dura Mater, that covers the fore-part of the Brain.

The Vertebral Artery in entring into the Skull, furnisheth it on each side with a considerable Branch, which is dispers'd throughout the whole Portion of the Dura Mater that covers the Cerebellum. {88}

As for the Veins that accompany these Arteries, they almost all go out of the Skull thro' the same Holes where the other enters.

There are four thick Arteries which convey to the Brain the Matter with which it is nourish'd, and that whereof the Spirits are form'd, viz. the two Internal Caroticks, and the two Vertebrals.

The Internal Carotick Arteries enter into the Skull thro a particular Ductus made in the Temporal Bone, the Mouth thereof being of an Oval Figure and situated in the outward part of the Basis of the Skull, before the Hole of the Internal Jugular. This Ductus extends it self obliquely from the back-side forward, and after having made about three Hairs breadth in length, is terminated in the hinder-part of the Os Sphenoides. The Artery traverseth the whole winding Compass of this Ductus, which resembles the Figure of the Roman Letter S, and at the Mouth of the same Ductus runs under the Dura Mater along the sides of the Os Sphenoides to the Anterior Apophyses Clinoides, where it riseth up again, to perforate the Dura Mater, and to adhere to the Root of the Brain. These Vessels, in like manner, after their departure from the Bone of the Temples to the place where they pierce the Dura Mater, make a second Circuit in form of the Roman Character S. At the place where these Carotick Arteries penetrate the Dura Mater, they send forth a thick Branch, which enters into the Orbit of the Eye, by the lower-part of the Hole, thro' which the Optick Nerve hath its Passage. {89}

The Vertebral Arteries proceeding from the Holes of the transverse Apophyses of the first Vertebra, turn about in passing under the upper oblique Apophyses of the seven Vertebra's: Afterward they perforate the Dura Mater, and running under the Marrow, enter into the Skull thro' the Occipital Hole; then inclining one toward another, they are re-united, and form only one single Trunk.

The Veins that bring back the Blood from the Substance of the Brain, are emptied into the Sinus's of the Dura Mater, which are all discharg'd into those that are call'd Lateral, which last go out of the Skull immediately under the Nerves of the eighth Pair, thro' the hinder-part of the Hole made by the meeting of the Occipital Bone, and the Apophysis Petrosa. These Lateral Sinus's fall into the Internal Jugulars, which are receiv'd into a considerable Sinking hollow'd on each side in the outward, part of the Basis of the Skull, which is nam'd the Pit or Hole of the Internal Jugular.

In the upper and hinder-part of the Hole, from whence the lateral Sinus's issue forth, is to be seen an opening in the Extremity of a Ductus, the Mouth whereof lies behind the Condyli, which are on the sides of the Occipital Trunk: This Ductus is extended about the length of two Hairs breadth in the Bone, and the Canal enclos'd therein is open'd immediately into the Vertebral Sinus: So that one might affirm it to be as it were its Original Source. Whence it appears that the Blood contained in the lateral Sinus's is emptied thro' two places; the greater Portion thereof descending in the Jugulars {90} from the Neck, and the other in the Vertebral Sinus's: Sometimes those Ductus's are four only on one side, another while both are stopt up, and the Blood contain'd in the lateral Sinus's is discharg'd into the Internal Jugulars.

Behind the Apophysis Mastoides on each side is a remarkable Hole, thro' which passeth a thick Vein, which brings back part of the Blood that hath been distributed to the Teguments and Muscles, which cover part of the Occiput or hinder-side of the Head: This Vein is open'd into the lateral Sinus's at the place where they begin to turn about. But in the Heads of some Persons, this Hole is found only on one side, and even sometimes not at all, in which case the Blood contain'd in the Vessels falls into the External Jugulars, with which the Branches of this Vein have a Communication.

In each Parietal Bone on the side of the Sagittal Suture, at a little distance from the Lambdoidal, appears a Hole, thro' which passeth a Vein, that brings back the Blood of the Teguments of the Head, and dischargeth it self into the upper Longitudinal Sinus. These Holes are sometimes on both; and then the Blood contain'd in the Branches of this Vein runs into the External Jugulars.

In the middle of the Sella of the Os Sphenoides, we may observe one or two small Holes thro' which (according to the Opinion of some Modern Anatomists) the Lympha contain'd in the Glandula Pituitaria is thrown {91} into the Sinus of the edge of the Os Sphenoides; nevertheless it is certain, that these Holes are fill'd only with Sanguinary Vessels, which carry and bring back the Blood of the Bones and Membranes, whereof those Sinus's are compos'd; besides that, these Holes are rarely found in adult Persons.

Between the Spine of the Coronal Suture and the Crista Galli, is a Hole which serves as an Entrance for a Ductus, which sinks from the top to the bottom, the length of about two Hairs breadth in the thickness of the inner Table of the Coronal: The Root of the upper Longitudinal Sinus is strongly implanted in this Hole, which also affords a Passage to some Sanguinary Vessels appointed for the Nourishment of this inner Table.

Many other small Holes are found in divers places of the Basis of the Skull; the chief whereof are those that are observ'd in the Apophysis Petrosa, and give Passage to a great number of Vessels that serve for the Nutriment of that part of the Temporal Bone which is call'd the Tympanum, or Drum: The other Holes are principally design'd for the Vessels that are serviceable in the nourishing of divers parts of the Basis of the Skull.

After what manner is the opening of the Head or Skull perform'd?

It is done by sawing it asunder round about and above the Ears; then it is taken off, after having before cut off the Hair, and made a Crucial Incision in the Skin from the fore-part to the hinder, and from one Ear to the other; as also after having {92} pull'd off and laid down the four Corners to the bottom.

How is the Brain anatomiz'd?

It is done by cutting it Superficially, and by Leaves, in order to discover by little and little the Ventricles, Vessels, and Nerves, with their Original Sources, &c. Or else it is taken entire out of the Skull, (the Nerves having been before examin'd) and laid down; so that without cutting any thing, all the parts of the Brain may be set in their proper places, to find out those that are sought for.

* * * * *

{93}

A

TREATISE

OF

Straps, Swathing-Bands, Bandages, Bolsters, Splints, Tents, Vesicatories, Setons, Cauteries, Leeches, Cupping-Glasses, and Phlebotomy.

* * * * *

CHAP. XVI.

Of Straps, Swathing-Bands, Bandages, and Bolsters.

What is a Strap?

It is a kind of Band commonly made use of for the Extension of the Members in the reducing of Fractures and Luxations; or else in binding Patients, when it is necessary to confine them, for the more secure performing of some painful Operation: These sorts of Ligatures have different Names, {94} according to their several Uses, and often bear that of their Inventer.

What is the Matter whereof these Straps are compos'd?

They may be of divers sorts, but are usually made of Silk, Wooll, or Leather.

What is a Swathing-Band?

It is a long and broad Band, that serves to wrap up and contain the Parts with the Surgeons Dressings or Preparatives.

Of what Matter are these Swathing-Bands made?

They are made at present of Linnen-Cloth but in the time of Hippocrates, were made of Leather or Woollen-Stuff.

How many sorts of Swathing-Bands are there in general?

There are two sorts, viz. the Simple and Compound; the former are those that are smooth, having only two ends; and the other are those which are trimm'd with Wooll, Cotton, or Felt, or that have many Heads, that is to say, Ends, fasten'd or cut in divers places according as different Occasions require.

What are the Conditions requisite in the Linen-Cloth, whereof the Swathing-Bands are made?

It must be clean, and half worn out, not having any manner of Hem or Lift.

What are the Names of the different Swathing-Bands?

There are innumerable, but the greater part them take their Denominations from their Figure or Shape; as the Long, Streight, Triangular, and those which have many Heads, or are trimm'd. {95}

What is A Bandage?

It is the Application of a Swathing-Band to any Part.

How many sorts of Bandages are there?

As many as there are different Parts to be bound; some of them being Simple, and others Compound: The former are those that are made with an uniform Band; as the Bandage call'd the Truss, and divers other sorts: The Compound are those that consist of many Bands set one upon another, or sew'd together; or else those that have many Heads. They have also particular Names taken from the Inventers of them, or from their Effect; as Expulsive Bandages to drive back, Attractive to draw forward, Contentive to contain, Retentive to restrain, Divulsive to remove, Agglutinative to rejoin, &c.

There are others whereto certain peculiar Names are appropriated; as Bridles for the lower Jaw, Slings for the Chin, the back part of the Head, Shoulder, and Perin 鵀 m; Scapularies for the Body, after the manner of the Scapularies of Monks; Trusses for Ruptures; Stirrups for the Ankle-Bones of the Feet, in letting Blood, and upon other Occasions. Lastly, there are an infinite Number of Bandages, the Structure whereof is learnt by Practice, in observing the Methods of able Surgeons, who invent them daily, according to their several Manners; and the first Ideas of these can only be taken in reading Authors that have treated of them.

What are the general Conditions to be observ'd in the Bandages? {96}

There are many, viz. 1. Care must be taken that the Bands be roll'd firm, and that they be not too streight nor too loose. 2. They are to be untied from time to time in Fractures, they must also be taken away every three or four Days, to be refitted. 3. They must be neatly and conveniently roll'd, that the Patient may not be uneasie or disquieted.

What ought to be observ'd in fitting the Bolsters?

Care must be taken to make them even, soft, and proportionable to the bigness of the Part affected; to trimm them most in the uneven places, that the Bands may be better roll'd over them, and to keep them continually moisten'd with some Liquor proper for the Disease as well as the Bands.

In treating of every Disease in particular, we shall shew the manner of making the particular Bandage that is convenient for it.

* * * * *

{97}

A

TREATISE

OF

Chirurgical Diseases.

* * * * *

CHAP. I.

Of Tumours in general, Abcesses or Impostumes, Breakings out, Pustules, and Tubercles.

What is a Tumour?

A Tumour is a rising or bloated Swelling rais'd in some part of the Body by a Setling of Humours.

How is this setling of Humours produc'd?

Two several ways, viz. by Fluxion and Congestion.

What is the Setling by Fluxion?

It is that which raiseth the Tumour all at once, or in a very little space of time, by the Fluidity of the Matter. {98}

What is the Setling by Congestion?

It is that which produceth the Tumour by little and little, and almost insensibly, by reason of the slow Progress and thickness of the Matter.

Which are the most dangerous Tumours, those that arise from Fluxion, or those that derive their Original from Congestion?

They that proceed from Congestion, because their thick and gross Matter always renders 'em obstinate, and difficult to be cur'd.

Whence do the differences of Tumours proceed?

They are taken, first, from the Natural Humours, Simple, Mixt, and Alter'd: Simple, as the Phlegmon, which is made of Blood, and the Erysipelas of Choler; Mixt, as the Erysipelas Phlegmon, which consists of Blood mingl'd with a Portion of Choler; or the Phlegmonous Erysipelas, which proceeds from Choler intermixt with a Portion of Blood: Alter'd, as the Melia which is compos'd of many Humours, that can not be any longer distinguish'd by reason of their too great Alteration. Secondly, the difference of Tumours is taken from their likeness to some other thing, as the Carbuncle and the Talpa, the former resembling a burning Coal, and the other a Mole, according to the Etymology of their Latin Names. Thirdly, From the Parts where they are situated; as the Ophthalmy in the Eye and the Quinsey in the Throat. Fourthly, from Disease that causeth 'em, as Venereal and Pestilential Buboes. Fifthly, from certain Qualities found in some, and not in others; as the Encysted Tumours, which have their Matter clos'd within their proper Cystes or Membranes, and so of many others. {99}

How many kinds of Tumours are there that comprehend at once all the particular Species?

They are four in Number, viz. the Natural Tumours, the Encysted, the Critical, and the Malignant.

What are natural Tumours?

They are those that are made of the four Humours contain'd in the Mass of the Blood, or else of many at once intermixt together.

What are the four Humours contain'd in the Mass of the Blood?

They are Blood, Choler, Phlegm, and Melancholy, every one whereof produceth its particular Tumour: Thus the Blood produces the Phlegmon, Choler the Erysipelas, Phlegm the Oedema, and Melancholy the Scirrhus. The Mixture of these is in like manner the Cause of the Erysipelatous Phlegmon, the Oedomatous Phlegmon or Phlegmonous Erysipelas, and the Phlegmonous Oedema, according to the quality of the Humours which are predominant, from whence the several Tumours take their Names.

What are the Encysted Tumours?

They are those the Matter whereof is contain'd in certain Cystes, or Membranous Bags; as the Meliceris, and the Struma or Kings-Evil.

What are Critical Tumours?

They are those that appear all at once in acute Diseases, and terminate them with good or bad Success.

What are Malignant Tumours?

They are those that are always accompany'd with extraordinary and dreadful Symptoms, and whose Consequences are also very dangerous; as the Carbuncle in the Plague. {100}

What are Impostumes or Abcesses, Breakings out and Pustules?

Indeed, it may be affirm'd, that all these kinds of Tumours scarce differ one from another, except in their size or bigness; nevertheless, to speak properly, by the Names of Impostumes or Abcesses are understood gross Tumours that are suppurable, or may be dissolv'd, and by those of Breakings out and Pustules, only simple Pusteal Wheals, or small Tumours, that appear in great Numbers, and which frequently do not continue to Suppuration; some of them consisting of very few Humours, and others altogether of dry Matter.

What difference is there between a Tumour and an Impostume or Abcess?

They differ in this particular, that all Tumours are not Impostumes nor Abcesses; but there is no Impostume nor Abcess that is not a Tumour: As for Example, Wens and Ganglions are Tumours, yet are not Abcesses nor Impostumes; whereas these last are always Tumours in regard that they cause Bunches and Elevations.

* * * * *

CHAP. II.

Of the general Method to be observ'd in the curing of Tumours.

What ought a Surgeon chiefly to observe in Tumours, before he undertake their Cure?

He ought to know three things, viz. 1. The Nature or Quality of the Tumour. 2. The {101} time of its formation and 3. Its situation: The Quality of the Tumour is to be known, because the Natural one is otherwise handl'd than that which is Encysted, Critical or Malignant. As for the time of its Formation, it is four-fold, viz. the Beginning, Increase, State, and Declination, wherein altogether different Remedies are to be apply'd. The Situation of the Tumour must be also observ'd, because the dressing and opening of it ought to be as exact as is possible, to avoid the meeting with an Artery or neighbouring Tendon.

How many ways are all the Tumours that are curable, terminated?

They are terminated after two manners, viz. either by dissolving 'em, or by

Suppuration.

Are not the Scirrhus and the Esthiomenus or Gangrene, two means that sometimes serve to terminate and cure Impostumes?

Yes, but it is done imperfectly, in regard that a Tumour or Impostume cannot be said to be absolutely cur'd, as long as there remains any thing of the Original Malady, as it happens in the Scirrhus, where the Matter is harden'd by an imperfect dissolving of it, or when the Impostume degenerates into a greater and more dangerous Distemper, as it appears in the Esthiomenus or Gangrene that succeeds it.

Which is the most effectual means of curing Impostumes, that of dissolving, or that of bringing them to Suppuration?

That of dissolving 'em is without doubt the most successful, and that which ought to be us'd as much as is possible; nevertheless some Cases are to be excepted, wherein the Tumours {102} or Abcesses are Critical and Malignant; for then the way of Suppuration is not only preferable, but must also be procur'd by all sorts of means, even by opening; which may be done upon this occasion, without waiting for their perfect Maturity.

What are the Precautions whereto a Surgeon ought to have regard before he undertake the opening of Tumours?

He must take care to avoid cutting the Fibres of the Muscles, and in great Abcesses, to cause all the corrupt Matter to be discharg'd at once, to prevent the Patient's falling into a Swoon.

Ought the opening of Tumours always to be made longitudinally, and according to the direct Course of the Fibres?

No, it is sometimes necessary to open 'em with a Crucial Incision, when they are large, or when a Cystis or Membranous Vehicle is to be extirpated.

How many sorts of Matter are there that issue forth in the Suppuration of Tumours?

There are four sorts, viz. the Pus, Ichor, Sanies, and Virus.

What isPus?

It is a thick Matter, and white as Milk.

What is Ichor?

It is a thick Matter like the Pus, but of divers Colours.

What is Sanies?

It is a watery Matter that riseth up in Ulcers, almost after the same manner as the Sap in Trees.

What is Virus? {103}

It is a kind of watry Matter, being whitish, yellowish, and greenish at the same time; which issueth out of Ulcers, very much stinking, and is endu'd with corrosive and malignant Qualities.

How many general Causes are there of Tumours?

There are three, viz. the Primitive, the Antecedent, and the Conjunct: The Primitive is that which gives occasion to the Tumours; as for Example, a Fall or a Blow receiv'd. The Antecedent is that which supplies it with Matter, such is the Mass of Blood that thickens and maintains the Phlegmon. Lastly, the Conjunct Cause is the overflowing Blood or Matter, which immediately forms the Tumor.

What regard ought to be had to these three sorts of Causes in the Cure?

The Primitive Cause may be prevented by avoiding the Falls, Blows, or other Hurts, and the Antecedent by diminishing the Plethory of the Blood, and cooling the whole Mass by Phlebotomy. The Conjunct Cause, which is the overflowing of the Blood, may be also remov'd in dispersing it by dissolving, or else in discharging it by Suppuration.

What is a Crisis?

It is a sudden setling of Humours, which happens in Diseases, whereby they are usually terminated.

How are these Critical Setlings effected?

By the Strength of Nature, which either expels the peccant Humours thro' the Belly, or carries them to the Habitude of the Body; for in the former she causeth Fluxes of Humours, Urine and Blood; as in the other she excites Sweatings, Tumours, and even a Gangrene it self.

In what Parts do the Critical Tumours usually arise? {104}

In the Glandules, which the Ancients call'd the Emunctories of the Brain, Heart, and Liver; for they gave the Name of Emunctories of the Brain to the thick Glandules which lie under the Ears, that of the Emunctories of the Heart to those that are under the Arm-Pits; and that of the Emunctories of the Liver to those under the Groin. Now Malignant Tumours may arise in all these parts, but the Venereal happen only in the Groin.

* * * * *

CHAP. III.

Of Natural Tumours.

* * * * *

ARTICLE I.

Of the Phlegmon and its Dependancies.

What is a Phlegmon?

It is a red Tumour occasion'd by the Blood diffus'd in some part, wherein it causeth extension, pain, and heat with beating.

Are Aneurisms and Varices, which are Tumours, made by the Blood, to be reckon'd among the Phlegmons?

No, because the Blood that forms the Aneurisms and Varices is not extravasated nor accompany'd with Inflammation, but only a Tumour of Blood proceeding from the Dilatation of the Arteries and Veins. {105}

May Echymoses or Contusions consisting of extravasated Blood, be esteem'd as Phlegmons?

By no means, in regard that it is not sufficient that the Blood be extravasated for the producing of a Phlegmon; it must also cause Pain, Heat, and a Beating, with Inflammation, which is not to be found in the Echymoses, except in great ones, after they have been neglected for a long time; where the corrupted Blood ought to be let out immediately, to prevent the Inflammation, overmuch Suppuration, and many other ill Consequences.

Is the Phlegmon always compos'd of pure Blood?

No, it may happen sometimes to partake of Choler, Phlegm, or Melancholy; on which account it is nam'd an Erysipelatous, Oedomatous, or Scirrhous Phlegmon, always retaining the Name of the predominant Humour, which is the Blood; and so of the others.

REMEDIES.

What are the Remedies proper for a Phlegmon?

They are of two sorts, viz. General and Particular; the former having regard to the antecedent cause, and the other to the conjunct. The Phlegmon is cur'd in its antecedent Cause, by Phlebotomy or letting Blood, by good Diet, and sometimes by Purgations, by which means the Plethory, Heat, and Alteration of the Blood is diminished; But Fomentations, Cataplasms and Plaisters facilitate the Cure in the conjunct cause, either by dissolving the Tumour, or bringing it to Suppuration. {106}

At what time is the Opening of a Vein necessary?

In the Beginning and Increase.

What are the Remedies proper to be us'd immediately upon the first appearing of the Tumour?

They are Resolvents and Anodynes; such as those that are prepar'd with Chervil boil'd in Whey, adding a little Saffron to wash the Tumour, and soak the Linnen Cloaths apply'd thereto, which are often renew'd, and may be laid on with the Chervil.

Or else take the Urine of a healthful Person, wherein is boil'd an Ounce of Saffron for a Glass, and bath the Tumour with it.

The Sperm of Frogs is also made use of to very good purpose, either alone, or with Lime-Water and Soap mixt together; or Oak-Leaves and Plantane beaten small, and apply'd. But Care must be more especially taken to avoid cooling Medicines, Oils, and Grease, which are pernicious in great Inflammations.

What ought to be done in the increase of the Tumour and Pain?

They are to be asswag'd by mollifying and dissolving; to which end a Cataplasm or Pultis is to be made with the Leaves of Elder, Wall-wort or Dwarf-Elder, Mallows, Violet-Plants, Camomile, and Melilot; whereto is added beaten Line-seed; causing the whole Mass to be boil'd in Whey, and allowing to every Pint, or thereabout, a Yolk of an Egg, twenty Grains of Saffron, a quarter of a Pound of Honey, and the Crum of white Bread, till it comes to a necessary Consistence. Or else take Cow's Dung instead of the above-mention'd {107} Herbs, and mix with it all the other Ingredients, to make a Cataplasm, which must be renew'd at least every twelve Hours.

What is to be done in the State?

If the Tumour cannot be dissolv'd (as was intended) it must be brought to Suppuration by Cataplasms, consisting of these Ingredients, viz. Garlick, White Lillies roasted under Embers, Milk, and Unguentum Basilicon.

Or else only take a Glass of Milk, in which an Ounce of Soap is dissolv'd, to wet the Linnen apply'd to the Tumour; and let it be often reiterated: Otherwise make use of Sorrel boil'd with fresh Butter, and a little Leaven or Yeast. The Plaister Diasulphuris is also most excellent either alone, or, if you please, mixt with Diachylon and Basilicon.

What is to be done in the Declination after the Suppuration?

The Ulcer must be at first gently dry'd with a Plaister of Diasulphuris or Diachylon, and afterward that of Diapalma may be us'd, and Ceruse or White Lead.

What Method is to be observ'd in case there be any Disposition toward a Gangrene?

It is requisite during the great Inflammation to make use of good Vinegar, in an Ounce whereof is dissolv'd a Dram of White Vitriol, with as much Sal Ammoniack, to bath the Tumour: Or else take the Tincture of Myrrh and Aloes, with a little Unguentum 茨 yptiacum, and afterward make a Digestive of Turpentine, the Yolk of an Egg, and Honey, mingling it with a little Spirit of Wine, or Brandy, if there remains any Putrifaction or Rottenness. {108}

Remedies for Aneurisms and Varices.

What is to be done in order to cure an Aneurism?

When it is little, as that which happens after an Operation of Phlebotomy or letting Blood ill perform'd, it may be sufficient to lay upon the affected Part a thin Plate of Lead, or else a Piece of Money or Counter wrapt up in a Bolster, and to bind it on very streight: But a Piece of Paper chew'd is much better for that purpose.

If the Anuerism be considerable, an Astringent Plaister may be us'd, such as the following.

Take Bolus, Dragon's Blood, Frankincence, Aloes, and Hypocystis, of each a Dram; mingle the whole with two beaten Eggs, and add Wax to give it the consistence of a Plaister, which may be apply'd alone, or mixt with an equal Portion of Emplastrum contra Rupturam, always making a small Bandage to keep it on. Emplastrum de Cicuta hath also a wonderful effect.

When the Aneurism is excessive, it is absolutely necessary to proceed to a Manual Operation, the manner whereof shall be shewn hereafter in the Treatise of great Operations.

What is requisite to be done in the Varices?

Varices are not generally dangerous, but even conduce to the preservation of Health; nevertheless, if they become troublesome by reason of their greatness, and the Pains that accompanie 'em, they may be mollify'd with the following Remedy.

Take the Mucilages of the Seeds of Psyllium and Line, of each two Ounces; of Populeon {109} two Ounces; Oleum Lumbricorum & Hyperici, of each one Ounce; and of the Meal of Wheat one Ounce, adding Wax to make the Consistence of a Plaister; part of which spread upon Linnen or Leather, must be apply'd to the Varix, and ty'd thereto with a small Band.

If the Blood abound too much, it may be discharg'd by the Application of Leeches, or by a Puncture made with a Lancet: Afterward lay upon the Part a Piece of Lead sow'd up in a Cloth, and let it be kept close with a proper Bandage. Otherwise you may make use of an Astringent, such as this.

Take a Pomegranate, cut it in pieces, and boil it with as much Salt as may be taken up with the Tip of your Fingers, in a Gallon of strong Vinegar; then dip a Spunge in this Vinegar, apply it to the Varix, bind it on, and continue the use of it twice a Day for a Month together.

Remedies for Echymoses, Contusions, or Bruises.

How are Echymoses to be treated?

All possible means must be us'd to dissolve 'em, by laying Slices of Beef upon the Part, renewing 'em very often, or applying Linnen Rags dipt in Spirit of Wine impregnated with Saffron.

They may be also dissolv'd with the Roots of Briony grated and apply'd thereto, or else with Plaister or Mortar, Soot, Oil of Olives and Unguentum Divinum, a Mixture whereof being made, is to be put between two Rags, and laid upon the Tumour or Swelling. {110}

If the Echymosis happens in a Nervous Part, Balsam of Peru may be us'd, or, for want thereof, Oleum Lumbricorum & Hyperici, with luke-warm Wine, with which the Bolsters must be soak'd, to be laid upon it.

When the Echymosis is great, and much Blood is diffus'd between the Skin and the Flesh, the safest way is to make an Opening to let it out, lest a too plentiful and dangerous Suppuration should ensue, or even a Gangrene it self. However, a Surgeon ought to proceed in the curing of an Echymosis in the Face with great Circumspection, which must be always prepar'd for Incision.

Of phlegmonous Tumors or Impostumes, and of Remedies proper for 'em.

What are the Tumours or Impostumes that partake of a Phlegmon?

They are the Bubo, Carbuncle, Anthrax, Furunculus, Phyma, Phygeton, Panaritium or Paronychia, Burn, Gangrene, and Kibe or Chilblain.

What is a Bubo?

A Bubo is a Tumour which ariseth in the Groin, being accompany'd with Heat, Pain, Hardness, and sometimes a Feaver.

What is a Carbuncle?

A Carbuncle is a hard Swelling, red, burning, and inseparable from a Fever: It is cover'd with a black Crust or Scab, that afterward falls off at the Suppuration, leaving a deep and dangerous Ulcer, and which sometimes doth not suppurate at all. {111}

What is an Anthrax?

The Anthrax is very near the same thing as the Carbuncle, only with this difference, that the latter always appears in the Glandulous Parts, and the Anthrax every where else.

What is a Furunculus?

It is a kind of Boil, or benign Carbuncle, which somewhat resembles the Head of a Nail, and is on that Account call'd Clou by the French, causing Pains, as if a Nail were driven into the Flesh.

What is a Phygeton?

The Phygeton is a small, red, and inflam'd Exuberance, situated in the Miliary Glandules of the Skin, where it causeth a pricking Pain, without Suppuration.

What is a Phyma?

The Phyma appears after the same manner as the Phygeton, and suppurates.

What are the Remedies proper for all these sorts of phlegmonous Tumours and Impostumes?

They are Cataplasms and Plaisters Anodyn, Emollient, Resolvent, and Suppurative, which are us'd proportionably as in the Phlegmons.

What is a Gangrene, Sphacelus, or Esthiomenus?

The Gangrene and Sphacelus signifie the same thing, nevertheless are commonly distinguish'd; the former being a Mortification begun, and the Sphacelus an entire or perfect Mortification; call'd also Necrosis and Sideratio. An Esthiomenus is a Disposition to Mortification, discover'd by the softness of the Part; and a Gangrene is defin'd to be a Mortification of a Part, occasion'd by the {112} Interception of the Spirits, and the Privation of the Natural Heat.

What are the causes of a Gangrene in general?

Every thing that can hinder the Natural Heat from exerting it self in a Part; as strong Ligatures, astringent or resolvent Medicines, not conveniently us'd in great Inflammations; a violent Hemorrhage; or Old Age, whereby the Spirits are exhausted; the bitings of Mad Dogs; excessive Cold, &c.

By what Signs is the Gangrene known?

It is discover'd by the livid Colour of the Skin, which departs from the Flesh, the softness, coldness, and insensibility of the Part; and sometimes by its dryness and blackness, from whence exhales a cadaverous Stench, with Sanies issuing forth after Punctures or Scarifications made therein. Lastly, a Gangrene is perceiv'd by the cold Sweats, Swoonings, Syncope's, and Delirium's that invade the Patient, and which are all the Fore-runners of approaching Death.

Is a Gangrene only found in the Flesh, and soft Parts of the Body?

It happens also in the Bones; and is then call'd Caries.

How is this Caries or Gangrene of the Bone discover'd, when it lies hid under the Flesh?

It is known by the black Colour of the Neighbouring Flesh, the Stink of the Sanies that comes forth, the intolerable Pains felt thereabouts, which are fix'd and continual before the Impostume and Ulcer appear; but when the Ulcer is made, a kind of roughness may be perceiv'd in the Bone. {113}

REMEDIES.

What are the Remedies proper for a Gangrene?

They are those that take away the mortify'd and corrupt Parts, and recall the Natural Heat; both which Indications are exactly answer'd in the Extirpation of what is already corrupted, with the Incision-Knife; and the Restauration of the Natural Heat by the following Remedies.

Take an Ounce of good Vinegar, steeping therein a Dram of White Vitriol, with as much Sal Ammoniack: Let it be us'd in bathing the Part; and apply thereto Bolsters well soak'd in the same Liquor. This Remedy is convenient in the first Disposition toward a Gangrene: Or, if you please, you may make use of the Yellow Water, which is made with Corrosive Sublimate and Lime-Water; taking, for Example, half a Dram of Corrosive Sublimate to be infus'd in a Pint of Lime-Water.

But a Tincture of Myrrh and Aloes is more efficacious, wherein Unguentum 茨 yptiacum is steep'd; or else Lime-Water kept for that purpose, in which have been boil'd two Ounces of Sulphur or Brimstone, with two Drams of Mercurius Dulcis; adding four Ounces of Spirit of Wine, to make an excellent Phegedick Water, with which the Part may be bathed, and the Bolsters soak'd.

If the Gangrene passeth to the Bone, the Ulcer must be immediately cleans'd with Brandy, and Euphorbium afterward put into it, laying also some upon the Bolsters, and {114} abstaining from all sorts of Oils and Greases. But if these Remedies prove unprofitable, recourse is then to be had to the Incision-Knife, Fire, or Amputation; the manner of performing which several Operations, is explain'd hereafter.

What are Kibes or Chilblains?

They are painful Tumours, which are often accompany'd with Inflammation; they happen more especially in the nervous and outward Parts, as the Heel, and are so much the more sensibly felt, as the Air and Cold are more sharp and Vehement.

What is to be done in order to cure these Kibes or Chilblains?

The Heel or affected Part must be wash'd and dipt in Wine boil'd with Allum and Salt, whereof a Cataplasm may be afterward made, by adding Meal of Rye, Honey, and Brimstone. The Juice of a hot Turnep apply'd with Unguentum Rosatum, is also very good, or Petroleum alone.

What is a Panaritium?

Panaritium or Paronychia, is a Tumour which generally ariseth in the Extremity of the Fingers, at the Root of the Nails: It is red, and accompany'd with very great Pain, even so exquisite, that the whole Arm is sensible thereof, insomuch that a Fever sometimes ensues, and a Gangrene; the Humour being contain'd between the Bone and the Periosteum, or that little Membrane with which it is immediately invested.

What Remedies are convenient for the curing of Panaritium? {115}

Anodyn Cataplasms are to be first apply'd, that is to say, such as serve to asswage excessive Pain, as that which is compos'd of Millk, Line-seeds beaten, large Figs, the Yolk of an Egg, Saffron, Honey and Oleum Lumbricorum, with the Crum of white Bread. Afterward you may endeavour to dissolve it, by applying Oil of Almonds, Saccharum Saturni, and Ear-Wax, or else Balsam of Sulphur. The Plaister of Mucilages, and that of Sulphur or Brimstone, dissolv'd in Wine, is also a most excellent Resolvent and Anodyn.

If it be requisite to bring this Tumour to Suppuration, white Lillies roasted under Embers may be added to the preceeding Cataplasm; or else a new Cataplasm may be made with Sorrel boil'd, fresh Butter, and a little Leaven.

What is a Burn?

A burn is an Impression of Fire made upon a Part, wherein remains a great deal of Heat, with Blisters full of serous Particles, or Scabs, accordingly as the Fire hath taken more or less effect.

What are the Remedies proper for a Burn?

A Burn is cur'd by the speedy Application of fresh Mud re-iterated many times successively; by that of peel'd Onions, Unguentum Rosatum, and Populeon, mixt with the Yolk of an Egg and unslack'd-Lime: Cray-Fishes or Crabs pounded alive in a Leaden-Mortar; and a great Number of other things.

If the Burn be in the Face, you may more especially take the Mucilages of the Seeds of Quinces and Psyllium, and Frog's-Sperm, of {116} each an equal quantity, adding to every four Ounces twenty Grains of Saccharum Saturni. This Composition may be spread on the Part with a Feather, and cover'd with fine Brown Paper. It is an admirable and approved Receipt.

If the Burn hath made an Escar or Crust, it may be remov'd with fresh Butter spread upon a Colewort or Cabbage Leaf, and apply'd hot. But in Case the Scab is too hard, and doth not fall off, it must be open'd, to give passage to the Pus or corrupt Matter, the stay of which would occasion a deep Ulcer underneath. The same Method is to be observ'd in the Pustules or Blisters, two Days after they are rais'd, applying also the Ointment of quick Lime, Oil of Roses, and Yolks of Eggs.

* * * * *

ARTICLE II.

Of the Erysipelas and its Dependances.

What is an Erysipelas?

An Erysipelas, commonly call'd St. Anthony's Fire, is a small Elevation produc'd by a Flux of Choler dispers'd and running between the Skin and the Flesh. It is known by its yellowish Colour, great Heat and Prickings.

REMEDIES.

What are the Remedies proper for an Erysipelas?

An Erysipelas that ariseth in the Head and Breast is not without danger, and the Cure of {117} it ought to be undertaken with great Care in the Application as well of internal as external Remedies: For it is requisite to take inwardly a Dose of the Diaphoretick Mineral, Crabs-Eyes, Egg-shels, Powder of Vipers, and other Medicines; as also Potions that have the like Virtues, such as the following. Take four Ounces of Elder-Flower-Water, adding thereto a Scruple of the volatile Salt of Vipers or Hart's-Horn with an Ounce of Syrrup of red Poppies.

Phlebotomy or Blood-letting hath no place here, unless there be a great Plethory, but frequent Clysters are not to be rejected, viz. such as are made of Whay, Chervil, Succory, and Violet-Plants, adding a Dram of Mineral Crystal dissolv'd with two Ounce of Honey of Violets.

As for outward Applications, Linnen-Rags dipt in the Spirit of Wine impregnated with Camphire and Saffron, are to be laid upon the Tumour, and renew'd as fast as they are dry'd. An equal quantity of Chalk and Myrrh beaten to Powder, may also be strew'd upon a Sheet of Cap-Paper over-spread with Honey, and apply'd to the Part.

If the Heat and Pain grow excessive, take half a Dram of Saccharum Saturni, twenty Grains of Camphire, as much Opium, with two Drams of red Myrrh, to be infus'd in a Gallon of White-Wine: Let this Liquor be kept to soak the Cloaths that are laid upon the Erysipelas, and often renew'd. But to dress the Face, a Canvass Cloth may be us'd, which hath been dipt in a Medicine prepar'd with a {118} Gallon of Whey, two Yolks of Eggs, and a Dram of Saffron.

Moreover amidst all these Remedies, it is necessary to oblige the Patient to keep to a good Diet, and to prescribe for his ordinary Drink a Diet-Drink made of Hart's-Horn, the Tops of the lesser Centory, Pippins cut in Slices with their Skins, and Liquorish; a little good Wine may be also allow'd, with the Advice of the Physician.

Of Erysipelatous Tumours or Impostumes, and their Remedies.

What are the Tumours or Impostumes that partake of the Nature of an Erysipelas?

They are the dry and moist Herpes, the former being that which is call'd the Tetter or Ring-Worm; and the other a kind of yellow-Bladders, Pustules, or Wheals, that cause itching, and raise small corroding Ulcers in the Skin: To these may be added divers sorts of Scabs and Itch.

The Remedies prescrib'd for the Erysipelas may be us'd for both these kinds of Herpes; as also Lotions or Bathing-Liquors made of Lime-Water, and a Decoction of Wormwood and Sal Ammoniack, allowing half a Dram to four Ounces of Liquor. Or else take half a Dram of Sal Saturni, and put it into a Glass of the Decoction of Fumitory or Chervil. You may also make use of the Oil of Tartar per deliquium, to make a Liniment either alone, or mingl'd with the above-mention'd Decoctions.

* * * * *

{119}

ARTICLE III.

Of the Oedema.

What is the Oedema?

It is a white soft Tumour, with very little sense of Pain, which ariseth from the Settling of a pituitous Humour.

What are the Remedies proper for an Oedema?

They are Fomentations, Cataplasms, Liniments, and Plaisters.

The Fomentations are made with Bundles of Wall-Wort or Dwarf-Elder, thrown into a hot Oven after the Bread is bak'd, and sprinkled with Wine: Afterward being taken out smoaking, they are unty'd, open'd, and wrapt about the Part, putting a warm Linnen Cloth over 'em. This Operation is to be re-iterated; and by this means the Humour is dissolv'd thro' Transpiration by Sweat.

The Cataplasms are compos'd of Camomile, Melilot, St. John's-Wort, Sage, Wall-Wort, Pellitory of the Wall, Roots of Briony and Onions, all boil'd together in White Wine with Honey, adding, if you please, a few Cummin or Fennel Seeds beaten. Cataplasms are also made of Horse-Dung and the Seeds of Cummin beaten, which are boil'd in strong Vinegar, and mixt with Barly-Meal to the Consistence of Pap.

The Plaisters are prepar'd with an Ounce of Diapalma, half on Ounce of Martiatum, a Pint of Oil of Lillies, half an Ounce of {120} Cummin-Seeds powder'd, half a Dram of Sal Ammoniack, and an Ounce of yellow Wax to make a Consistence.

If any hardness remains, the Plaister of Mucilages may be apply'd, or that which is made of the Gums Bdellium, Ammoniack, and Galbanum, dissolv'd in Vinegar. But Care must be taken not to omit the Purgatives of Jalap to the quantity of a Dram in a Glass of White-Wine; or of half an Ounce of Lozenges of Diacarthamum, which are effectual in drawing out the bottom of pituitous and serous Humours that nourish the Oedema's.

Of Oedomatous Tumours and Impostumes.

What are the kinds of Tumours that partake of the Nature of an Oedema?

They are the Phlyctea, the Emphysema, the Batrachos or Ranunculus, the Wen, the Talpa, the Bronchocele, the Ganglion, the Fungus, the Scurf, the Scrophula or King's-Evil, and all sorts of Dropsies both general and particular.

What are Phlyctea's?

They are Pustules or Blisters fill'd with a white and somewhat yellowish Humour.

What is an Emphysema?

It is a kind of flatuous Tumour, wherein Wind is contain'd, with a little slimy Phlegm.

What is a Batrachos or Ranunculus?

It is a Blister fill'd with slimy Water, that ariseth under the Tongue near the String, and in French is call'd Grenouillette, or the little Frog; which is the same with its Greek and Latin Names. {121}

What is a Wen?

It is a Tumour consisting of thick plaistry Phlegm, which is reckon'd among the Encysted.

What is a Talpa?

It is a soft and very broad Tumour, which usually appears in the Head and Face, containing a white, thick and pituitous Matter.

What is a Bronchocele?

It is a bunch'd Tumour which ariseth in the Throat, and causeth it to swell extremely; being compos'd of thick Phlegm mix'd with a little Blood, and ranked among the Encysted Tumours.

What is a Ganglion?

It is a very hard Tumour, void of Pain and wavering, produc'd by thick Phlegm: But it is always found upon some Nerve or Tendon.

What is a Fungus?

It is a spungy Tumour that grows upon Tendons bruis'd or weaken'd by some Hurt.

What is the Scurf?

It is a whitish and scaly Tumour rais'd in the Skin of the Head by a viscous and mixt Phlegm, having its Root in the bottom of the Skin.

What is the Scrophula or King's-Evil?

Scrophul?or Strum? commonly call'd the King's-Evil, are Tumours that generally shew themselves in the Glandules of the Neck, and in all those Parts where there are any. They consist of a viscous, serous, and malignant Phlegm, The Source or Root whereof is suppos'd to be in the Glandules of the Mesentery. They are also of the number of the Encysted Tumours. {122}

What is the Dropsie?

It is a soft Tumour occasion'd by the setling of abundance of serous Matter in the Parts where it appears.

How many sorts of Dropsies are there?

There are three general Species, viz. the Ascites, Tympanites, and Leucophlegmatia.

What is an Ascites?

It is a kind of Dropsy that forms the Tumour or Swelling of the Abdomen or lower Belly, by a Mass of Water.

What is a Tympanites?

It is a kind of Dropsy, which in like manner causeth a Tumour or Swelling in the lower Belly, with this difference, that a great deal of Wind is mixt with the Water, which renders the Tumour transparent, and sounding, as it were a Drum; whence this Disease hath taken its Name.

What is the Dropsy call'd Leucophlegmatia?

It is a Tumour, or, to speak more properly; a general Swelling or Bloating of all the other Parts of the Body, as well as of the lower Belly. It is produc'd by a viscous and mucilaginous sort of Phlegm; whence it happens that the Print of the Fingers remains in those places that have been press'd.

What are the particular kinds of Dropsies?

They are those that are incident to different Parts, of which they bear the Names; as the Hydrocephalus, which is the Dropsy of the Head; the Exomphalus, of the Navel, and the Hydrocele of the Scrotum. There is also a Dropsy of the Breast, and that of the Matrix.

{123} What are the Remedies proper for all these sorts of Tumours or Dropsies?

They are in general all those that are agreeable to the Oedema, which are variously us'd, as Liniments, Fomentations, Cataplasms, and Plaisters: Internal Medicines ought also to be much consider'd, as Diaphoreticks, Sudorificks, and Purgatives, when they are assisted by a regular Diet.

A Decoction of the Roots of Briony with Cinnamon and Liquorish, provokes Urine very much; as well as a Decoction of Turneps and Carrets, and an Infusion of Sage in White-Wine.

* * * * *

ARTICLE IV.

Of a Scirrhus, and its peculiar Remedies.

What is a Scirrhus?

It is a hard unmoveable Tumour, almost altogether void of Pain, and of a livid dark Colour; which is form'd of a Melancholick Humour, frequently succeeding Phlegmons and Oedema's that have not been well dress'd with convenient Remedies.

How is a Scirrhus cur'd?

By mollifying or dissolving it, and seldom by bringing it to Suppuration.

It may be mollify'd by the application of a Cataplasm or Pultis, compos'd of the Leaves of Violet-Plants, Mallows, Beets, Elder, Rue, and Wormwood, with Camomile-Flowers, {124} Horse-Dung, Cow-Dung, and White Lillies. The whole Mass is to be boil'd together in Wine, afterward adding Honey and Hogs-Lard, to make a Cataplasm thereof with the Crum of White Bread.

It is dissolv'd with Plaisters compos'd of those of Diachylon, Melilot, and Mucilages, to which is added Oleum Lumbricorum, and Flower of Brimstone. To render the Remedy more effectual, Oil of Tobacco may be also mixt with it, and Gum Ammoniack dissolv'd in Vinegar.

Furthermore, these Topical or outward Medicines are to be accompany'd with others taken inwardly, which serve to prepare the Humours for convenient Evacuations; Such are Crab's-Eyes, the Decoctions of Sarsaparilla, the use of good Wine, and light Meats of easie Digestion.

Of Scirrhous Tumours, and their Remedies.

What are the Tumours that partake of the Nature of a Scirrhus?

They are the Polypus, Carcinoma, Sarcoma, Natta, and Cancer.

What is a Polypus?

It is an Excrescence of fungous Flesh arising in the Nostrils: But Hippocrates confounds the Carcinoma and Sarcoma with the Polypus, of which he says they are only a Species.

What is the Natta?

It is a Tumour or Excrescence of Flesh that appears in the Buttocks, Shoulders, Thighs, Face, and every where else, the various Figures {125} of which cause it to be call'd by different Names. For one while it resembleth a Gooseberry, at another time a Mulberry, and at another time a Melon or Cherry. Sometimes also these Swellings are like Trees, Fishes, Birds, or other sorts of Animals, according to the ardent desire that Women with Child have had for things that they cou'd not obtain when they longed for 'em.

What are the Remedies proper for the Polypus, and other kinds of Excrescences of the like Nature?

The Polypus may be cur'd in the beginning, but it is to be fear'd lest it degenerate into an incurable Cancer, when it hath been neglected or ill dress'd.

Besides the general Remedies, which are letting Blood a little, and reiterated Purgations, with an exact Regulation of Diet, there are also particular Medicaments which dry up and insensibly consume the Excrescence; as a Decoction of Bistort, Plantain, and Pomegranate-Rinds in Claret-Wine, which is to be snuff'd up the Nose many times in a Day, and serves to soak the small Tents that are put up therein, as also often to cool the Part, adding a little Allum and Honey.

The Patient must sometimes likewise keep in his Mouth a Sage-Leaf, sometimes a piece of the Root of Pellitory of Spain; and at another time Tobacco or some other thing of this Nature, which causeth Salivation. If the Tumour continues too long, and doth not yield to the above-mention'd Remedies, it is necessary to proceed to a Manual Operation, {126} which is very often perform'd with good Success.

As for the Natta's, it is most expedient not to meddle with 'em at all; nevertheless these Marks which Infants bring along with 'em into the World, are frequently defac'd by an Application of the After-Burdens, whilst they are as yet warm, as soon as their Mothers are deliver'd.

What is a Cancer?

It is a hard, painful, and ulcerous Tumour, produc'd by an adult Humour, the Malignity whereof can scarce be suppress'd by any Remedies.

How many sorts of Cancers are there?

There are two kinds, viz. The Primitive and the Degenerate; the Primitive Cancer is that which comes of it self, and appears at first about the bigness of a Pea or Bean, which nevertheless doth not cease to cause an inward Pain, continual, and pricking by intervals; during this time it is call'd an Occult Cancer; but when grown bigger, and open'd, it bears the Name of an Ulcerated Cancer; which is so much the less capable of being cur'd or asswag'd, as it makes it self more conspicuous by its dreadful Symptoms, or concomitant Circumstances.

The Degenerate Cancer is that which succeeds an obstinate and ill-dress'd Tumour or Impostume, and which becomes an Ulcerated Cancer, without assuming the Nature of a blind or occult one.

What Remedies are requisite to be apply'd to a blind Cancer? {127}

In regard that it cannot be known in this Condition without difficulty, it is often neglected; nevertheless it is a Matter of great Moment to prevent its Consequences, more especially by a good Diet, and by general Remedies, which may gently rectifie the intemperature of the Bowels: Afterwards Baths may be prescrib'd, together with the use of Whey Asses-Milk, and Specificks in general, as Powders of Crab's Eyes, Vipers, Adders, and others. As for Topical Remedies, none are to be administer'd, except it be judg'd convenient to apply to the Tumour a Piece of Lead rubb'd with Quick-silver; all others serving only to make the Skin tender, and apt to break. The Patient may also take for his Drink Water of Scorzonera and Hart's-Horn, with the Flowers of Bugloss or Borage, and Liquorice: Or else Quick-silver-Water alone, boiling an Ounce of it in a Quart of Water every time, the Quick-silver always remaining at the bottom of the Vessel.

What are the Remedies for an ulcerated Cancer?

Besides the general ones, that are the same with those of the blind Cancer, there are also Topical, which may take place here. The Powders of Toads, Moles, Frogs, and Crabs calcin'd, cleanse the Ulcers perfectly well. A Decoction of Vipers and Crabs may serve to bath 'em, and some of it may be taken inwardly. Detersives made of Lime-Water, or Whey clarify'd, and boil'd with Chervil are very good; and (if you please) you may add Camphire or Saccharum Saturni. {128}

If the Pains grow violent, recourse is to be had to Laudanum, one or two Grains whereof may be given in a little Conserve of Roses. When the Cancer is situated in the Glandules or Flesh, the Extirpation of it may also be undertaken with good Success.

As for the manner of handling Degenerate Cancers, respect must be always had to the kind of Tumour, from whence it deriv'd its Original.

* * * * *

CHAP. IV.

Of Bastard or Encysted Tumours.

What is an Encysted or Bastard Tumour or Impostume?

It is that which is made of a Setling of mixt and corrupt Humours, the Matter whereof is contain'd in certain proper Cystes or Membranous Bags.

What are the kinds of these Tumours?

They are the Steatoma, the Atheroma, the Meliceris, the Wen, the Bronchocele, and the Scrophula or King's-Evil.

How is the difference between these Tumours discern'd?

The Steatoma is known by its Matter resembling Suet; as that of the

Atheroma resembleth Pap; and that of the Meliceris is like Honey: These three Tumours cannot be well distinguish'd on the outside, in regard that they do not change the natural Colour of the Skin, which {129} equally retains in all three the print of the Fingers that press it. But the Bronchocele is discover'd by the Place and Part which it possesseth; that is to say, the Throat; as also by its somewhat hard consistence without the Alteration of the Skin. The Scrophul?or King's-Evil Swellings are known by their unequal Hardness, and their situation in the Glandules, either in the Neck, Arm-pits or elsewhere, without alteration likewise of the Skin.

REMEDIES.

Want is the Method to be observ'd in curing these sorts of Tumours?

An Attempt is to be made to dissolve 'em, as in all the others; nevertheless the safest way is to bring 'em to Suppuration, and to extirpate the Cystes, which are apt to be fill'd again after the Dissipation of the Humour.

What are the Medicines proper to dissolve these Tumours?

They are all such as may be us'd for the Oedema and Scirrhus; but the Specificks or particular Remedies are these:

Take Rosemary, Sage, Wormwood, Elder, great Celandine, Camomile, Melilot, St. John's-Wort, and Tobacco; boil 'em in White-Wine with Soot and Mercurial Honey, adding, thereto Cummin-seeds beaten, and Oleum Lumbricorum, to make a Cataplasm, which is to be renew'd twice a Day. Afterward if the Tumour be not dispers'd, you may apply the following Plaister, which hath an admirable Effect. {130}

Take an equal Portion of the Plaister of Diachylon, Devigo, and four times as much Mercury, and Emplastrum Divinum; let 'em be dissolv'd together; then intermix Saffron, and Oil of Tobacco, to make a Plaister with the whole Mass, which may be spread upon thin Leather, and apply'd to the Tumour, without taking it off only once every eighth Day, to cool it; so that it must be laid on again after having wash'd and bath'd the Part with warm Urine or Brine.

But it is to be always remember'd that external Remedies take effect only imperfectly, unless they are assisted by internal, such as in this case are reiterated Purgations, join'd with a regular Diet.

What are the Remedies proper to excite Suppuration?

To this purpose those may be us'd that serve in other kinds of Tumours: But as for the extirpation of the Cystis, it is done by dividing the Tumour into four Parts, by procuring Suppuration, and by consuming the Bag by little and little. The Bronchocele alone will not admit this Extirpation, by reason of the great Number of Nerves, Veins, and neighbouring Arteries amidst which the Tumour is settl'd. However Bronchotomy, or opening the Throat, may be perform'd; which is an Operation peculiar to this Tumour.

* * * * *

{131}

CHAP. V.

Of Critical, Malignant, Pestilential, and Venereal Tumours and Impostumes.

What difference is there between Critical, Malignant, Pestilential, and Venereal Tumours?

It consists in these particular circumstances, viz. that Critical Tumours or Impostumes are indifferently all such as are form'd at the End or Termination of Diseases, in whatsoever Place or Part they appear.

Malignant Impostumes or Tumours are those that are obstinate, and do not easily yield to the most efficacious Remedies.

Pestilential Impostumes or Tumours are those that are accompany'd with a Fever, Swooning, Head-ach, and Faintness: They usually arise in the time of a Plague or Pestilence, and are contagious.

Venereal Tumours or Impostumes are those that appear only at the bottom of the Groin, and are the product of an impure Coitus.

However, the Critical Impostume may be Malignant, Pestilential, and Venereal; the Malignant Impostume may be neither Critical, nor Pestilential, nor Venereal: But the Pestilential and Venereal Tumours are always Malignant. {132}

What are the ordinary kinds of Critical Tumours or Impostumes?

They are the Anthrax, the Boil, the Phlegmon, and the Parotides or Swellings in the Almonds of the Ears.

What are the kinds of Malignant Tumours or Impostumes?

They are the Cancer, the Scrophula or King's-Evil; and others of the like Nature.

What are the kinds of Pestilential Tumours or Impostumes?

They are Carbuncles that break out every where; a sort of Anthrax which appears under the Arm-pits, and Bubo's in the Groin.

What are the kinds of Venereal Tumours or Impostumes?

They are Botches or Bubo's and Cancers that arise in the Yard; as also Wens and Condyloma's in the Fundament.

What is the difference between a Pestilential and a Venereal Buboe?

They may be distinguish'd by their Situation, and respective Accidents; the Pestilential lying higher, and the Venereal lower: Besides, a Fever, Sickness at the Heart, and an universal Faintness or Weakness, are the ordinary concomitant Circumstances of the former; whereas the Venereal Buboe is always the consequence of an impure Coitus, and is attended with no other Symptoms than those of common Tumours, viz. Pain, Heat, Shootings or Prickings, &c.

As for the Remedies, they may be sought for among those that have been already prescrib'd for Tumours.

* * * * *

{133}

CHAP. VI.

Of the Scurvy.

This Disease is known by the Ulcers of the Mouth, which are very stinking; as also by excessive Salivation, great Pains in the Head, Dizziness, frequent Epilepsies, Apoplexies, and Palsies. The Face, being of a pale red, and dark Colour, is sometimes puff'd up or bloated, inflam'd, and beset with Pustules: The Teeth are loose and ake, the Gums are swell'd, itch, putrifie, exulcerate, and are eaten with the Canker; and the Jaw is almost unmoveable: The Members are bow'd, and cannot be extended: The Patients become stupid and drowsie, so that they fetch their Breath with difficulty, are obnoxious to Palpitations of the Heart and Coughs, and fall into Swoons: The Ulcers sometimes are so malignant, that their Cheeks are entirely eaten up, and their Teeth seen: They are also much inclin'd to Vomitting, Looseness, and Gripes; and their Entrails are swell'd: They have red and livid Pustules on their Belly and Privy-parts, which sometimes break out into Ulcers; their whole Body being dry'd, &c.

This Disease may be easily cur'd in the beginning; but when it is grown inveterate, and invades the Bowels, it becomes incurable; as well as when it is the Epidemical Disease of {134} the Country, or the Persons afflicted with it, are old, or well advanc'd in Years.

In undertaking the Cure, it is requisite to begin with a good Diet, and to sweeten the Blood, let the Patient take the Broth of boil'd Fowl; eating Pullets and Eggs; in the Broth may also be put divers sorts of Antiscorbutick Herbs; viz. Cresses, Spinage, Parsly-Roots, Sparagus, Smallage, Scorzonera, Scurvy-Grass, &c. Let him eat nothing that is high season'd, nor acid or sharp; let him drink pure Claret, without any adulterate Mixture; let him use moderate Exercise and Rest; Lastly, let him keep his Mind sedate, and free from all manner of violent Passion.

The following Remedies taken inwardly are very good for the Scurvy, viz. the

Tincture of Flints from ten Grains to thirty; Diaphoretick Antimony, from six Grains to thirty; sweet Sublimate, from six Grains to thirty; Mars Diaphoreteus, from ten Grains to twenty; Crocus Martis Aperitivus, from ten Grains to two Scruples; prepar'd Coral, from ten Grains to one Dram; Volatile Spirit of Sal Ammoniack, from six Drops to twenty; Water of Cresses, from fifteen Drops to one Dram; Spirit of Scurvy-grass, from ten Drops to one Dram; Tincture of Antimony, from four Drops to twenty; Oily Volatile Sal Ammoniack, from four Grains to fifteen; Spirit of Guyacum, from half a Dram to a Dram and a half; Vitrioliz'd Tartar, from ten Grains to thirty; the Volatile Salt of Tartar, Urine, Vipers, and Hart's-Horn, of each from six Grains to fifteen; the Spirit of Gum Ammoniack, from eight Drops to sixteen; White {135} Mercury Precipitate, from four to ten Grains; Mercurial Panacea, from six Grains to two Scruples. We shall shew the manner of compounding 'em in our Treatise of Venereal Diseases.

It is also expedient to give Emollient and Detersive Clysters to the Patient at Night going to bed, his Body being always kept open with convenient Diet-drinks: Afterward let him take gentle Sudorificks, such as are made of the Decoctions of Fumitory, wild Cicory, Dandelion, Hart's-Tongue, Scabious, the lesser House-Leek, Germander, Borage, Scorzonera-Root, and Polypody, with Flowers of Broom, Elder, and Marygold.

These are stronger for cold Constitutions, viz. Decoctions of Scurvy-Grass, Lepidium, Arse-smart, the lesser Celandine, Wormwood, little House-Leek, Trifolium Febrinum, Angelico, Juniper-Berries, &c.

Convenient Decoctions to wash the Mouth may be made with Sage, Rosemary, Hyssop, Oak-Leaves, Scurvy-Grass, Cresses, Tobacco, Roots of Bistort, Aristolochy or Birth-Wort, Tormentil, Flower-de-Luce, Balaustia or Pomegranate-Flowers, Red Roses, &c.

To corroborate the Gums, Gargarisms are made of Anti-Scorbutick Plants; as of Spirit of Scurvy-Grass two Drams, one Scruple of Spirit of Vitriol, one Scruple of common Salt, four Ounces of Rose-Water and Plantane-Water. But if the Gums are putrefy'd, they are to be rubb'd with Honey of Roses, and some Drops of Spirit of Salt.

To asswage the Pains of the Members, Bathings and Fomentations are to be us'd; and a {136} Decoction of Saxifrage taken inwardly, with some Grains of Laudanum is good for that Purpose.

To allay the Gripes, Clysters may be given with Whey, Sugar, Yolks of Eggs, Syrrop of Poppies, and Oils of Earth-Worms, Scurvy-Grass, Camomile, &c.

Against the Scorbutick Dropsy, take the Essence of Trifolium Febrinum and Elicampane, from twenty four Drops to thirty, and continue the use thereof.

Milk taken inwardly hinders Vomitting; and a Broth or Gelly of Crabs sweetens the Blood. The Looseness may be stopt with the Essence of Wormwood, and Spirit of Mastick; as also the Fever with Febrifuges and Antiscorbuticks.

The Spots may be fomented with Decoctions of Aromatick and Anti-Scorbutick Herbs and Nitre. For the Ulcers of the Legs, pulverize an equal quantity of Saccharum Saturni, Crocus Martis, Myrrh, and Mercurius Dulcis, and lay it upon the Bolsters that are to be apply'd to the Sores.

To mollifie the sharpness of Acid Humours, this is a good Remedy: Prepare half an Ounce of Spirit of Scurvy-Grass, two Drams of tartariz'd Spirit Ammoniack, a Dram of the Tincture of Worms. Take thrice a Day fifteen or twenty Drops of this Liquor, in a Decoction of the Tops of Firr.

Against the Tubercles, take two Handfuls of the Flowers of Camomile and Elder, three Drams of Briony-Root, and an Handful of White-Bread Crum; Boil the whole Composition in Milk, and make Cataplasms thereof. {137}

To mitigate the Pains in the Head, take twenty or thirty five Drops of the Tincture of Amber, in Anti-scorbutick Spirits or Waters.

The difficulty of Respiration may be remov'd by a Medicinal Composition made of two Drams of an Anti-scorbutick Water, two Drams of the Essence of Elicampane, and half a Dram of the Spirit of Gum Ammoniack; take three or four Spoonfuls thereof several times in a Day.

To prevent the putrefaction of the Gums, take one Dram of the Tincture of Gum Lacca, three Drams of the Spirit of Scurvy-Grass, with fifteen or twenty

Drops of Oil of Tartar made per Deliquium, and rub the Gums with this Composition many times in a Day. Brandy in which Camphire is infus'd, or Spirit of Wine, is likewise a most excellent Remedy; as also all Lotions or Washes made with the Waters or Decoctions of Anti-scorbutick Plants.

For Leanness, Goat's-Milk with the Spirit of Scurvy-Grass may be us'd, and other Waters drawn from Anti-scorbutick Plants. The Apozemes or Decoctions of Endive, Cicory, Sorrel, Becabunga, and Snail-Water, are in like manner very good for the same purpose.

Ointment of Styrax is frequently us'd in the Hospital call'd Hotel-Dieu at Paris, and apply'd to Spots and callous Swellings that arise in the Legs.

* * * * *

{138}

A

TREATISE

OF

Wounds, Ulcers, and Sutures.

* * * * *

CHAP. I.

Of Sutures.

Sutures or Stitches are made only in recent, and as yet bleeding Wounds, when they cannot be re-united by Bandage, as are the transverse; provided there be no Contusion, nor loss of Substance, nor great Hemorrhages, as also that the Wounds were not made by the biting of venomous Beasts, that there be no violent Inflammations, and that the Bones are not laid open; because generally 'tis necessary to cause 'em to be exfoliated; neither is this Operation to be perform'd in the Breast, by reason of its Motion.

The Instruments proper for the making of Stitches, are streight and crooked Needles, {139} with waxed Thread; and these Sutures are of four sorts, viz. first the Intermittent Stitch for transverse Wounds; the second for the Hare-Lip; the third, commonly call'd the Dry Stitch, for superficial Wounds; and the fourth, term'd the Glover's Stitch.

The Intermittent Stitch is that which is made at certain separated Points, according to the following manner: After having taken away all extraneous Bodies out of the Wound, let a Servant draw together its Sides or Lips; and let a Needle with waxed Thread be pass'd thro' the middle from the outside to the inside, several Points being made proportionably to its length. It is requisite to pierce a good way beyond the Edge of the Wound, and to penetrate to the bottom, lest any Blood shou'd remain in the Space, that might hinder the reuniting.

If the Wound hath Corners, the Surgeon begins to sow there; and before the Knot is made, causeth the Lips of the Wound to be drawn exactly close one to another: The Knots must be begun with that in the middle, and a single one is first made on the side opposite to the running of the Matter; laying upon this Knot (if it be thought convenient) a small Bolster of waxed Linnen, on which is tied a Slip-Knot, to the end that it may be untied if any bad Accident should happen. If a Plaister be apply'd to the Wound after the Stitching, a small Bolster is to be laid over the Knots, to prevent their sticking to the Plaister. In case any Inflammation happens in the Wound, the Knots may be loosen'd and ty'd again when the Symptoms cease: But {140} if the Inflammation continue, the Threads are to be cut by passing a Probe underneath: When the Wound is clos'd, the Threads are cut in like manner with a Probe; and in drawing 'em out, a Finger must be laid near the Knot, lest the Wound should open again.

To make the second sort of Stitch for the Hare-Lip, a small streight Needle is pass'd into the sides of the Wound, and the Thread is twisted round the Needle, by crossing it above at every Stitch.

To form the Dry Stitch in very superficial Wounds, a piece of new Linnen-Cloth is to be taken, wherein are made Digitations, or many Corners; the Selvedge or Hem ought to be on the side of these Corners or Digitations; and a small Thread-Lace is ty'd to every one of 'em. Afterward this Cloth is dipt in strong Glue, and apply'd about a Finger's breadth from the Edges of the Wound; so that a piece thereof being stuck on each side, the Laces may be ty'd together, to cause the Lips of the Wound to meet.

To make the Glover's Stitch, the Operator having drawn together the Lips of the Wound, holds 'em between two Fingers, passeth a Needle underneath 'em, and soweth 'em upward all along, after the manner of Glovers.

* * * * *

{141}

CHAP II.

Of Wounds in general.

What is a Wound?

A Wound is a recent, violent, and bloody Rupture or Solution of the Natural Union of the soft Parts, made by a pricking, cutting, or bruising Instrument.

What ought to be observ'd before all things in the curing of Wounds?

It is requisite to take notice of their differences, as well as of the Instruments with which they were made; to the end that Consequences may be drawn from thence for the Application of proper Remedies.

From whence arise the differences of Wounds, and which be they?

They are taken either from their Figure or Situation: With regard to their Figure, they are call'd Long, Broad or Wide, Triangular Great, Little, Superficial, or Deep; and with respect to their Situation, they are term'd Simple, Complicated, Dangerous, or Mortal.

What is a Simple and a Complicated Wound?

A Simple Wound is that which only opens the Flesh, and hath no other concomitant Circumstances; but a Complicated Wound, on the contrary, is that which is attended with grievous Symptoms, as Hemorrhages, Fractures of Bones, Dislocation, Lameness, and others of the like Nature. {142}

What is a dangerous and mortal Wound?

A dangerous Wound is that which is complicated the Accidents whereof are dreadful: As when an Artery is open'd or prick'd, when a Nerve or Tendon is cut, or when the Wound is near a Joynt and accompanied with a Dislocation or Fracture. A mortal Wound is that which must be inevitably follow'd by Death; as is that which is situated deep in a principal Part necessary for the Preservation of Life.

What are the Parts wherein Wounds are mortal?

They are the Brain, the Heart, the Lungs, the Oesophagus or Gullet, the Diaphragm, the Liver, the Stomach, the Spleen, the small Guts, the Bladder, the Womb, and generally all the great Vessels.

Wherein doth the Cure of Wounds consist?

In helping Nature readily to procure the reuniting of the Parts that have been divided, after having taken away or asswag'd every thing that might cause an Obstacle.

What are the things that hinder the speedy reunion of the Parts?

They are extraneous Bodies found therein, as Bullets, Flocks, and Pieces of Wood or Stone, &c. As also sometimes the Accidents which attend 'em; as an Hemorrhage or Flux of Blood, Inflammation, Esthiomenus or Mortification, Hypersarcosis, or an Excrescence of Flesh, Dislocation, the Fracture of a Bone, the Splinter of a Bone, & sometimes a contrary Air. {143}

REMEDIES.

What are the Remedies proper for stopping an Hemorrhage or Flux of Blood?

The common Remedy is a kind of Cataplasm, made up with the Powders of Aloes, Dragons-Blood, Bole Armenick and Whites of Eggs, which are mix'd together and laid upon the Wound. But the following is an excellent one.

Take two Ounces of Vinegar, a Dram of Colcothar, two Drams of Crocus Martis Astringens; beat the whole together, steeping Muscus Quercinus therein; then throw upon it the Powder of Mushrooms, or of Crepitus Lupi: Apply this Remedy, and you'll soon stop the Hemorrhage, taking Care nevertheless to bind the Part well, otherwise the Astringents do not readily take Effect.

To this Purpose you may also make use of Cobwebs, Mill-Dust, and the Powder of Worm-eaten Oak; or else take Oven-Soot mixt with the Juice of the Dung of an Ass or Ox, adding only thereto the White of an Egg.

Besides these Remedies there are also actual and potential Cauteries, or simple Ligatures, which are infallible. Indeed the actual Cautery is not always sure; because when the Escar made by the Fire, falls off the Hemorrhage breaks out again as before: but the potential Cautery is almost always successful; such as the following.

Take about an equal Quantity of Vitriol and Powder of Mushrooms; apply 'em upon a little Lint to the Place where the Blood issueth {144} forth, and you'll see it stop immediately: But Care must be taken to avoid touching a Nerve or Tendon; by reason that the Vitriol is apt to excite Convulsions.

How is the Inflammation and Mortification of a Wound Suppress'd?

If the Inflammation proceeds from the Presence of an Extraneous Body, it must be taken away as soon as possible with a Pair of Forceps, and if from the Quantity of Pus or corrupt Matter, it must be let out. But in case the Inflammation ariseth from extreme Pains, they are to be asswaged with Cataplasms or Pultises and anodyn Liniments, such as those that have been already prescribed in the Cure of the Phlegmon: or else the Part may be bath'd with Camphirated Spirit of Wine, mixt with as much Water: Saccharum Saturni infus'd in Lime-water, performs the same Effect, and the Water of Crabs alone is admirable in its Operation.

Against the Esthiomenus or Mortification, make use of Wine boil'd with Wormwood, St. John's Wort, Rosemary and Aloes; or else take the Tincture of

Aloes and Myrrh, or Spirit of Wine alone impregnated with Camphire and Saffron.

What is to be done in Case a Convulsion happens by reason of a wounded Nerve or Tendon?

If the Convulsion be caus'd by the Presence of an Extraneous Body that bruiseth the Part it must be taken away; and if from the wounding of a Nerve, pour into the Wound some Drops of the Oil of Lavender distill'd, which in that Case is of singular Use; this Oyl may be also taken inwardly in an appropriated Liquour, such as a {145} Decoction of Wormwood and the Tops of the lesser Centory. Balsam of Peru us'd in the same Manner, is an excellent Remedy, and the Oyls of Worms, Snails, St. John's-Wort and Turpentine are frequently apply'd with good Success.

If the Convulsion proceeds from the Biting of some venomous Creature, Cupping-Glasses or Leeches are to be immediately applied, putting into the Wound Treacle with the Spirit of Wine or even Fire it self, and leaving to the Physician's Care the Prescription of other vulnerary Remedies proper to be taken inwardly.

What is to be done to draw the Extraneous Bodies out of a Wound?

When they cannot be taken away with the Fingers or Forceps, the Patient must be set in the same Station or Posture wherein he was when he receiv'd the Wound, in order to get some farther Light to discover 'em; or else such Plaisters may be us'd as are endu'd with an Attractive Quality: Particularly this:

Take an Ounce of Treacle, half a Dram of Gum Ammoniack, one Dram of Bdellium, and two Drams of Bore's Grease, adding a Quarter of a Pound of Wax to make 'em up into the Form of a Plaister. It is reported that Hare's Grease alone hath the same Effect, and that it goes for a Secret among the Surgeons but you may (if you please) mix it with Ointment of Betony. However it hath been observed that Leaden Bullets may sometimes remain in a Man's Body, during his whole Life-time without doing any Harm. {146}

How are Excrescences to be taken away?

They may be consum'd with Powder of Allom, Unguentem or Lapis infernalis.

After having remov'd every thing that hinders the reuniting of the Lips of a Wound, what is to be done to attain thereto?

The Re-Union in Wounds is properly the Work of Nature; but it may be promoted by putting into 'em a little Balsam of Peru, and drawing together their Lips with the Fingers. Afterwards the Lips must be kept closed with a Bandage, a Glutinous Plaister or a dry Stitch, provided the Wound be only superficial, hindring the Air from penetrating into it. For Want of Balsam of Peru, an excellent one may be made with the Flowers here specified.

Take the Flowers of Henbane, St. John's-Wort, and Comfry and let 'em be digested in the Sun during the whole Summer-Season in the Oyl of Hemp-seed, which Oyl, the longer it is kept, proves so much the better, if it be set forth in the Sun every Summer, the Vessel that contains it being well stop'd. There is also the Balsam of Balsams, or the Balsam of Paracelsus call'd Samech.

To avoid the exposing of Wounds to the Air, it is requisite to cover 'em over the Dressings with some sort of Plaister, which is usually termed the Surgeon's Plaister, such is that which is effectual in Dissolving, corroborating and allaying Pain or Inflammation.

Take the Mucilages of the Roots of great Comfrey and Fenegreek, half a Pound of Ceruse or white Lead, two Drams of Crude Opium, one Dram of Camphire, as much of Saffron, two Drams of Sandarack, one of the Oyl of {147} Bays, one half Pound of Rosin, and as much Turpentine and Wax. Boil all these Ingredients together in a sufficient Quantity of Lin-seed-Oyl, and make a Plaister according to Art.

In great Wounds it is expedient to lay over the Dressings a Cataplasm or Pultiss, such as this:

Take the Leaves and Flowers of Camomile, and Melilot, the Tops of Wormwood, common Mallows and Marsh-Mallows, with the Seeds of Line and Cummin powder'd: Then boyl the whole Composition in Wine, and add thereto Barly-Meal, to give it a due Consistence. If there be any Cause to fear a Gangrene, you may also intermix Saffron, Myrrh and Aloes with Spirit of Wine.

Is it necessary to put Tents into all Wounds, and to make use of Digestives and Suppuratives?

No: It is sufficient to procure the Re-uniting of the Parts simply by the Means of Balsam in small Wounds; because they ought not to be brought to Suppuration: so that Digestives and Suppuratives are only necessary in great Wounds, and those that are accompanied with Contusion, avoiding the ill Custom of some Country-Surgeons, that stuff up their Wounds too much with Tents and Pledgets, whereas they might well be content with simple Bolsters or Dossels which shou'd be dipt in the ordinary Digestive composed of Turpentine and the Yolks of Eggs with a little Brandy, or else with the Tincture of Myrrh and Aloes.

Suppuration may also be promoted by mundifying and quickening the Wound, especially if the Bolsters be steep'd in the following Composition. {148}

Take half an Ounce of Aloes and Myrrh powder'd, two Drams of Sal Saturni, twenty Grains of Sal Ammoniack, the same quantity of beaten Cloves, a Dram of Queen of Hungary Water and half an Ounce of Unguentum Basilicon, and let the whole Mass be mingled together.

In fine, the whole Mystery consists in well cleansing the Wounds with a Linnen Cloth, or with the Injections of the Tinctures of Myrrh and Aloes; or with simple Decoctions of Wormwood, Scordium or Water-Germander, Bugle, Sanicle and Hore-Hound in White-Wine; as also by prescribing the Vulnerary Decoctions of Powder of Crab's-Eyes, and Saccharum Saturni, to be taken inwardly, to consume the acid Humours, which are a very great Obstacle that hinders the speedy cure of Wounds.

What are the Vulnerary Plants, the Decoctions of which is to be taken inwardly?

They are Alchymilla or Lion's-Foot, Ground-Ivy, Veronica or Fluellin, St. John's-Wort, Wormwood, Centory, Bugle, Sanicle, Chervil, and others. The

Broth of Crabs may also be prescrib'd, which is an excellent Remedy, and may serve instead of a Vulnerary Potion.

Sometimes Sutures or Stitches contribute very much to the re-uniting of the Lips of Wounds, when they cannot be join'd by Bandage.

* * * * *

{149}

CHAP. III.

Of particular Wounds of the Head.

What ought first to be consider'd in a Wound of the Head?

Two things, that is to say, the Wound it self, and the Instrument with which it was made; for by the Consideration of the Wound, we may know whether it be Superficial or Deep; and by that of the Instrument, we are enabled to make a truer Judgment concerning the Nature of the same Wound.

What is a Superficial, and what is a Deep Wound in the Head?

That is call'd a Superficial Wound in the Head, which lies only in the Skin; and that a Deep one which reacheth to the Pericranium, Skull, or Substance of the Brain.

What is to be apply'd to a Superficial Wound?

It is cur'd with a little Queen of Hungary Water; or else with a little Balsam, laying upon it the Surgeon's Plaister, or that of Betony. But if the Wound or Rent be somewhat large, it must be clos'd with a Stitch.

What is to be done to a Deep Wound?

If it be situated in the Pericranium, the Wound must be kept open, waiting for Suppuration; but if it enter the Skull, an Enquiry is to be made, whether there be a Simple Contusion, or a Fracture also. In the Contusion it is necessary to wait for the Suppuration, and the {150} fall of the Splint, and to keep the Wound open; as in the Fracture, to examine whether it be in the first Table only, or in both; it is known to be only in the first, by the Application of an Instrument, and of Ink, as also in regard that there are no ill Symptoms; but a Fracture in both Tables shews it self by the Signs; and it may be found out by making a Crucial Incision in the Flesh, to discover the Fissure.

What are the Signs of the Fracture of the two Tables of the Skull, and of the overflowing of the Blood upon the Membranes of the Brain?

They are the loss of the Understanding at the very Moment of receiving the Wound; an Hemorrhage or Flux of Blood thro' the Nose, Mouth, or Ears; drowsiness and heaviness of the Head, and more especially Vomitting of Phlegm; from whence may be inferr'd the necessity of making use of the Trepan.

What Consequence may be drawn from the Knowledge of the Instrument with which the Wound was made?

It is according to the Quality of this Instrument; as it is proper to cut, prick, or bruise; if it be cutting, the Wound is more Superficial, and not subject to a great Suppuration: If it be pricking, the Wound is deeper, but of small Moment: If it be a battering or bruising Instrument, the Wound is accompany'd with Contusion, producing a great Suppuration, besides the Concussion and Commotion of the Part, which are inseparable, and often cause very dangerous Symptoms. {151}

Inferences may be made also from the disposition of the wounded Person; for a strong robust Man may better bear the Stroke than a weak one; and even Anger causeth an Augmentation of Vehemency; so that all such Circumstances are not to be despis'd, in regard that they give occasion to profitable Conjectures.

What particular Circumstance is there to be observ'd in undertaking the Cure of Wounds in the Face?

It is, that a more nice Circumspection is requir'd here than elsewhere, in abstaining from Incisions, as well as in making choice of proper Medicines, which must be free from noisome Smells; and it is in this Part chiefly that Balsams are to be used, avoiding Suppuration, to prevent Scars and other Deformities.

* * * * *

CHAP. IV.

Of the particular Wounds of the Breast.

What is to be observ'd in Wounds of the Breast?

Two things, viz. whether they penetrate into the Cavity of the Thorax or not, which may be discover'd by the Probe, and by a Wax-Candle lighted, and apply'd to the Entrance of the Wound, obliging the Patient to return to the same Posture wherein he receiv'd the Hurt, as also to keep his Nose and Mouth shut: For then the Flame may be perceiv'd to be wavering, the Orifice of the Opening being full of {152} Bubbles; a Judgment may be also made from the running out of the Blood.

What is to be done when it is certainly known that the Wound penetrates into the Cavity of the Breast?

It is necessary to examine what Part may be hurt, by considering the situation of the Wound, and its Symptoms: If the Lungs are pierc'd, a spitting of froathy Vermilion-colour'd Blood ensues, with difficulty of Respiration, and a Cough. If any of the great Vessels are open'd, the wounded Person feels a Weight at the bottom of his Breast, is seiz'd with cold Sweats, being scarce able to fetch his Breath, and Vomits Blood, some Portion whereof issueth out of the Wound. If the Diaphragm or Midriff be cut in its Tendinous Part, he is suddenly hurry'd into Convulsions: And if the Heart be wounded either in its Basis or Ventricles, he falls into a Swoon, and dies incontinently.

But if the Probe doth not enter, and none of the above-mentiond Symptoms appear, it may be taken for granted that the Wound is of no great Consequence.

What is to be done when the Wound penetrates into the Chest, yet none of the Parts are hurt, only there is an Effusion of Blood over the Diaphragm?

It is necessary to make an Empyema, or otherwise the diffus'd Blood in corrupting, wou'd inevitably cause an Inflammation, Gangrene, and Death it self.

What is an Empyema?

It is an Operation whereby any sorts of Matter are discharg'd with which the Diaphragm is over-spread, by making a Puncture or Opening in the Breast.

* * * * *

{153}

CHAP. V.

Of the particular Wounds of the lower Belly.

What is to be done to know the quality of a Wound made in the lower Belly?

It is requisite to make use of the Probe, to observe the situation of the Wound, and to take notice of all the Symptoms: For by the help of the Probe, one may discover whether it hath penetrated into the Cavity or not, after having enjoyn'd the Patient to betake himself to the same Posture wherein he was when he first receiv'd the Wound: By its situation a Conjecture may be made that such a particular Part may be hurt; and by a due Examination of the Symptoms, one may attain to an exact Knowledge. As for Example; It is known that one of the thick Guts is open'd, when the Hurt is found in the Hypogastrium, and the Excrements are voided at the Wound; as it is certain that one of the thin Guts is pierc'd, when the Wound appears in the Navel, and the Chyle issueth forth from thence; and so of the others.

What Method ought to be observ'd in curing Wounds in the lower Belly?

It is expedient at first to prevent letting in the Air, and to dilate the Wound, in order to sow up the perforated Gut, and afterward to {154} restore it to its place; as also to bind the Caul, which is let out at the opening, and to cut it off, lest in putrifying it should corrupt the neighbouring Parts. Then these Parts may be bath'd with Lees of Wine, wherein have been boil'd the Flowers of Camomile and Roses with Wormwood: The Powders of Aloes, Myrrh, and Frankincense may be also thrown upon 'em; and the Wound must be sow'd up again to dress it on the outside, the Patient in the mean time being restrain'd to a regular Diet. But Clysters must be forborn on these Occasions, especially when one of the thick Guts is wounded, making use rather of a Suppository or laxative Diet-Drinks, to avoid dilation and straining.

* * * * *

CHAP VI.

Of Wounds made by Guns or Fire-Arms.

These Wounds are always bruis'd and torn, with the loss of Substance, and commonly with the splitting and breaking of a Bone: They are red, black, livid, and inflam'd, not being usually accompany'd with an Hemorrhage: They are generally round, and streighter at their Entrance than at their End; at least if they were not made with Cross-Bar-Shot, or Quarter-Pieces. {155}

Of the Prognostick of Wounds by Gun-shot.

When these Wounds penetrate into the Substance of the Brain, or Marrow of the Back-Bone, or into the Heart, Pericardium, great Vessels, and other noble Parts, Death always inevitably follows, and often happens at the very Instant. But one may undertake the Cure of those that are superficial, and which are made in the Neck, Shoulders, Arms, and all other parts of the Body.

Of the Cure of Wounds by Gun-shot.

For the better curing of these sorts of Wounds, it is requisite to be inform'd of the Quality of the Fire-Arms by which the Wounds were made, in regard that a Musquet is more dangerous than a Pistol, and a Cannon much more than a Musquet; as also to examine their situation and concomitant Accidents; for by how much the more complicated they are, so much the greater is the danger. Then the Patient must be set (as near as can be) in the very same Situation and Posture wherein he remain'd when the Wound was receiv'd, in order to discover the direct Passage of the Wound by the help of the Probe, with which a search is to be made, whether a Bullet, or any other extraneous Bodies, as Wood, Flocks, Linnen, or Stuff as yet stick in the Wound; so that Endeavours may be us'd to take 'em out thro' the same Hole where they enter'd, care being more especially had to avoid making {156} Dilacerations in drawing 'em out: But if the Operator hath endeavour'd to no purpose to remove these extraneous Bodies, let him make a Counter-Opening in the opposite Part, where he shall perceive any hardness, nevertheless without touching the Vessels; thus the Incision being made, he may readily draw 'em out with his Fingers, or some other Instrument.

If the Bullet sticks so far in a Bone that it cannot be taken away without breaking the same Bone, it is more expedient to let it lie therein; but if the Leg or Arm-Bones are very much split or shattered, then the Amputation of 'em becomes absolutely necessary. The Pain and Inflammation of the Part may be asswag'd by letting Blood, topical Anodyns, cooling Clysters and Purgations; but in case much Blood hath been already lost, Phlebotomy must be omitted. The Clysters may be made with Decoctions of Mercury, Mallows, Beets, a Handful of Barley and Honey of Roses.

Some Surgeons are of Opinion that the Patient ought to be purg'd every other Day, and even on the very same Day that he receiv'd the Wound, if his Strength will permit; however very gentle Purges are to be us'd upon this occasion, such as Cassia, Manna, Tamarins, Syrrup of Violets, and that of White Roses.

In the mean while Anodyns may be compounded to mitigate the Pain; as Cataplasms or Pultisses made with the Crum of white Bread, Milk, Saffron, the Yolk of an Egg, and Oil of Roses us'd hot; which last Ingredient is of it self a very good Anodyn. But to asswage great Inflammations, Oil of {157} Roses, the White of an Egg and Vinegar beaten all together, may be laid on the neighbouring Parts.

At first it is necessary to apply spirituous Medicines to the Wound, and Pledgets steep'd in camphirated Brandy, are admirable for that purpose; but if there be a Flux of Blood, styptick Waters, or other astringent Remedies may be us'd, still remembering that all these Medicaments must be apply'd hot.

To promote the Suppuration of these contused Wounds, a Digestive may be made of Oleum Rosatum, the Yolk of an Egg, and Venice Turpentine.

If the Wound be in the Nerves, Tendons, or other Nervous Parts, it is requisite to use spirituous and drying Medicines, never applying any Ointments, which will not fail to cause Purtrefaction in those Parts: But a Cataplasm may be made with Barley-Meal, Orobus, Lupins and Lentils boil'd in Claret, adding some Oil of St. John's-Wort.

The Balsam of Peru, Oil of Turpentine destill'd, Oil of Wax, destill'd Oil of Lavender, Oleum Philosophorum, Oil of Bays destill'd, Balsam of St. John's-Wort, Spirit of Wine, and Gum Elemi, are excellent Medicaments for the Nerves: Or else,

Take four Ounces of Unguentum Alth 骀 with a Dram and a half of destill'd Bays; mingle the whole Composition, and apply it: Or else,

Take an Ounce of destill'd Oil of Turpentine, a Dram of Spirit of Wine, and half an Ounce of Camphire; let all be intermixt, and dropt into the Wound: Or else, {158}

Take a Scruple of Euphorbium, half an Ounce of Colophonia, and a little Wax; let 'em be mingl'd together, and apply'd very hot to the Nervous Parts.

If the Wounds are deep, Injections may be made with this Vulnerary Water, which is very good for all sorts of Contusions, as also for the Gangrene and Ulcers.

Take the lesser Sage, the greater Comfrey, and Mugwort, of each four Handfuls; Plantane, Tobacco, Meadowsweet, Betony, Agrimony, Vervein, St. John's-Wort, and Wormwood, of each three Handfuls; Fennel, Pilewort Bugle, Sanicle, Mouse-Ear, the lesser Dazy, the lesser Centory, and All-heal, of each three Handfuls; three Ounces of round Birth-Wort, and two Ounces of long: Let the whole Composition be digested during thirty Hours, in two Gallons of good White-Wine, and afterward destill'd in Balneo Mari? till one third part be consumed.

If a Gangrene happens in the Part, Spirit of Mother-Wort may be put into it, which is compounded with two Drams of Mastick, Myrrh, Olibanum, and Amber, and a Quart of rectify'd Wine, the whole being destill'd.

This Fomentation may be apply'd very hot to very good purpose, viz. an equal quantity of Camphirated Wine and Lime-Water, with three Drams of Camphire.

This is also an excellent Cataplasm: Take a Pint of Lye, and as much Spirit of Wine, half an Handful of Rue, Sage, Scordium, and Wormwood, a Dram of each of the Roots of both sorts of Birth-Wort, and two Drams of {159} Sal Ammoniack. Let the whole Composition be boil'd till a third Part be consum'd; adding half a Dram of Myrrh and Aloes, and a little Brandy.

Of a Burn made by Gun-Powder.

If the Burn be recent, and the Skin not exulcerated, Spirit of Wine or Brandy is to be immediately apply'd; or else an Ointment may be made with Oil of Olives, or bitter Almonds, Salt, the Juice of Onions, and Verjuice.

If the Skin be ulcerated, and little Bladders or Pustules arise, an Ointment may be compounded with the second Bark of Elder boil'd in Oil of Olives. After it hath been strain'd, add two parts of Ceruse or White-Lead, and one of Burnt Lead, with as much Litharge, stirr'd about in a Leaden-Mortar, to make a Liniment. But it is not convenient to take out the Grains of Powder that remain in the Skin, because they are apt to break, and to be more confounded or spread abroad; so that they must be left to come forth in the Suppuration.

When the Wound is superficial, and the Skin as yet whole, peel'd Onions with common Honey are an excellent Remedy; but if the Skin be torn, it is not to be us'd, by reason that the Pain wou'd be too great; in which case Oil of Tartar per diliquium hath a very good effect.

If the Burn be accompany'd with a Fever, it may be allay'd with fixt Nitre, Nitre {160} prepar'd with Antimony, and Gun-Powder taken inwardly, which are very effectual in their Operation. Crab's-Eyes prepar'd, and even some of 'em unprepar'd, are in like manner admirable Remedies.

As for external Medicaments, when the Burn is only superficial, take Onions and unslack'd Lime, quench'd in a Decoction of Rapes, and apply this Liquor very hot, with double Bolsters dipt therein. Or else take what quantity you please of quick Lime well wash'd, and pound it thoroughly in a Leaden-Mortar, with May-Butter without Salt, to make an Ointment, which may be laid altogether liquid upon the affected Part: Or else,

Take as much quick Lime as you can get up between your Fingers at two several times; Milk-Cream and clarify'd Honey, of each about half the like quantity; let the whole be intermix'd to the Consistence of an Ointment, and apply'd: It is an approv'd Remedy; as also is the following;

Take unslack'd Lime, and put it into common Water, so as the Water may appear four or five Finger's breadth above it. After the Effervescence, pour in Oil of Roses; whereupon the whole Mass will be coagulated in form of Butter, and may be apply'd.

A good Lotion or Washing-Liquor may be prepar'd with the Juice of Garlick and Onions, in recent Burns; otherwise make use of this Ointment. Take an Ounce and an half of raw Onions, Salt, and Venice Soap, of each half an Ounce; mingle the whole Composition in a Mortar, pouring upon it a sufficient {161} quantity of Oil of Roses, to make a very good Ointment: Or else,

Dissolve Minium or Litharge in Vinegar, filtrate this Liquor, and add thereto a quantity of Rape-Oil newly drawn off, sufficient to give it the Consistence of a liquid Liniment; then stir it about in a Leaden-Mortar till it become of a grey Colour, and keep it for Use as an excellent Liniment: Or else,

Pound Crey-Fishes or Crabs alive in a Mortar to get their Blood, and foment the Part with it hot; it is a good Remedy: Otherwise intermix the pounded Crabs with May-Butter without Salt, and let 'em be boil'd up together, and scumm'd, till a red Ointment be made, which may be drawn off, or strain'd for Use. And indeed, all manner of Ointments, and other Medicinal Compositions wherein Crabs are an Ingredient, are true specificks against Burns made by Gun-Powder.

The Mucilages of the Seeds of Psyllium, or rather those of Quince-Seeds prepar'd with Frog's Sperm, and a little Saccharum Saturni, spread with a Feather upon the affected Part, have a wonderful Operation in Burns.

A Medicament compounded with one third part of the Oil of Olives, and two of the Whites of Eggs well beaten and mixt together, is a very simple and singular Remedy. Otherwise take half an Ounce of Line-seed-Oil infus'd in Rose-Water, with four Yolks of Eggs; beat 'em together, and let the whole be apply'd to the burnt Part.

If the Burn be very violent, and hath many Pustules, Etmullerus is of Opinion that they {162} ought to be open'd, and that an Ointment shou'd be apply'd, which is made of Hen's-Dung boil'd in fresh Butter: Otherwise,

Take a handful of fresh Sage-Leaves, two handfuls of Plantane, six Ounces of fresh Butter without Salt, three Ounces of Pullet's-Dung newly voided, and the whitest that can be found; then fry the whole Composition for a quarter of an Hour; squeeze it out, and keep it for use: Otherwise,

Take two Ounces of sweet Apples roasted under Embers, Barly-Meal, and Fenugreek, of each half an Ounce, and half a Scruple of Saffron; let the whole Mass be mingled to make a Liniment or soft Cataplasm, which may serve to asswage Pain, and mollifie the Skin.

If the Wound be yet larger, and hath a Scab, open all the Pustules, and endeavour the two first Days to cause the Escar to fall off by the Application of a Liniment made of the Mucilages of Quince-Seeds steept in Frog's-Sperm, with fresh Butter, the Oil of White Lillies, and the Yolk of an Egg: Otherwise,

Make a Liniment with fresh Butter well beaten in a Leaden-Mortar, with a Decoction of Mallows, which being spread upon hot Colewort-Leaves, and apply'd to the Escar, it will fall off.

But if the Escar be too hard and obstinate, it is requisite to proceed to Incisions to make way for the Sanies, lest a deep and putrid Ulcer shou'd be engender'd Underneath. As soon as the Humour is evacuated, the above-mention'd {163} Emollient Medicines may be us'd, till the separation of the Escar; then the Ulcer may be consolidated with Digestives and Mundificatives; such as the Ointment of quick Lime with Oil of Roses, and the Yolks of Eggs.

The white camphirated Ointments, and that of Alabaster, are also good for the same Purpose.

If a Gangrene ensueth, Sudorificks must be taken inwardly; such are camphirated Spirit of Treacle, the Essence and Spirit of Elder-Berries, the Spirit of Hart's-Horn with its own proper Salt, Treacle impregnated with the Spirit of camphirated Wine, Scorpion-Water, Hart's-Horn, Citron with Camphire, &c.

As for external Remedies in the beginning of the Gangrene, the Spirit of Wine apply'd hot is excellent; and yet better if Aloes, Frankincense, and Myrrh be intermixt therein. It ought also to be observ'd, that Camphire must always be mingled in the topical Medicines for the Cure of the Gangrene.

A Decoction of unslack'd lime, in which Brimstone hath been boil'd, with Mercurius Dulcis, and the Spirit of Wine, is a very efficacious Remedy.

In a considerable Gangrene, after having made deep Scarifications, let Horse-Dung be boil'd in Wine, and laid upon the Part in form of a Cataplasm. This is an approved Remedy.

If a Sphacelus be begun, scarifie the Part, and apply thereto abundance of Unguentum 灸 yptiacum over and above the Ointments and Cataplasms already describ'd; remembring {164} always, that when the Gangrene degenerates into a Sphacelus, all the mortify'd Parts must be incontinently separated or cut off from the sound.

* * * * *

CHAP. VII.

Of Ulcers in general.

What is an Ulcer?

An Ulcer is a Rupture of the Natural Union of the Parts made a long while ago, which is maintain'd by the Sanies that runs out of its Cavity; or an Ulcer takes its Rise from a Wound that cou'd not be well cur'd in its proper time, by reason of the ill quality of its Pus or corrupt Matter.

What difference is there between a Wound and an Ulcer?

It is this, that a Wound always proceeds from an external Cause, and an Ulcer from an internal, such as Humours that fall upon a Part; or else a Wound in growing inveterate degenerates into an Ulcer.

Whence is the difference of Ulcers deriv'd?

It is taken from the Causes that produce 'em, and the Symptoms or Accidents with which they are accompany'd. Thus upon Account of their Causes they are call'd Benign or Malignant, Great, Little, Dangerous, or Mortal; and by reason of their Accidents, they are term'd Putrid, Corrosive, Cavernous, Fistulous, Cancerous, &c. {165}

Do Ulcers always proceed from external Causes, or from an outward Wound degenerated?

No they sometimes also derive their Origine from internal Causes, as the Acrimony of Humours, or their Malignant Quality; the Retention of a Splint of a Bone, and other things of the like Nature. These Ulcers are commonly call'd Primitive, and the others Degenerate.

What are Putrid, Corrosive, Cavernous, Fistulous and Cancerous Ulcers?

The Putrid Ulcer is that wherein the Flesh is soft and scabby, the Pus and Ichor being viscous, stinking, and of a cadaverous smell.

The Corrosive Ulcer is that which by the Acrimony and Malignity of its Sanies, corrodes, makes hollow, corrupts and mortifies the Flesh.

The Cavernous Ulcer is that the Entrance of which is streight and the bottom broad wherein there are many Holes fill'd with malignant Sanies, without any callosity or hardness in its sides.

The Fistulous Ulcer is that which hath long, streight, and deep Holes, with much hardness in its sides; the Sanies whereof is sometimes virulent, and sometimes not.

The Cancerous Ulcer is large, having its Lips bloated, hard, and knotty, of a brown Colour, with thick Veins round about, full of a livid and blackish sort of Blood. In the bottom are divers round Cavities, which stink extremely, by reason of the ill Quality of the Sanies that runs out from thence.

Are there no other kinds of Ulcers? {166}

Yes, there are also Verminous, Chironian, Telephian, Pocky, Scorbutick, and others, which have much affinity with, and may well be reckon'd among the five Kinds already specify'd.

What are the means to be us'd in the curing of Ulcers?

Ulcers ought to be well mundify'd, dry'd and cicatriz'd; but with respect to the several Causes and Accidents that render 'em obstinate, and difficult to be cur'd, it is also requisite to make use of internal Medicines, which may restrain and consume 'em. If their sides grow callous, they are to be scarify'd, in order to bring 'em to Suppuration; and if there be any Excrescences, they must be eaten away with corroding Powders, such as that of Allom; or by the Infernal Cautery.

What are the Remedies proper to cleanse and dry up Ulcers?

To this Purpose divers sorts of Liquors may be us'd, as also Powders and Plaisters: The Liquors are usually made of Briony-Roots, the greater Celandine, Lime, and Yellow Water; a Tincture of Myrrh, Aloes and Saffron, and Whey, whereto is added Saccharum Saturni; so that the Ulcers may be wash'd or bath'd with these Liquors; and very good Injections may be compounded of 'em.

The Powders are those of Worm-eaten-Oak, Allom, and Cinoper, the last of these being us'd by burning it, to cause the Fume to be convey'd to the Ulcer thro' a Funnel. The Country People often make use of Potter's-Earth to dry up their Ulcers, with good {167} Success; but then they must must be of a Malignant Nature.

The Plaisters are Emplastrum de Betonica, Diasulphuris, Dessiccativum Rubrum, and others; and the Ointments are such as these;

Take three Yolks of Egg, half an Ounce of Honey, and a Glass of Wine, and make thereof a mundifying Ointment, according to Art: Otherwise,

Take Lime well wash'd and dry'd several times, let it be mingled with the Oil of Line and Bolus, and it will make an excellent Ointment to mundifie and dry; a little Mercury Precipitate may be intermixt (if you please) to augment the drying Quality; and Mercurius Dulcis may be added in the Injections.

For Ulcers in the Legs, and Cancerous Ulcers, take Plantain-Water and Allom-Water, or else Spirit of Wine, Unguentum 灾 yptiacum, and Treacle; or else an Extract of the Roots of round Birth-Wort made in the Spirit of Wine. Gun-Powder alone dissolv'd in Wine, is of singular Use to wash the Ulcers, and afterwards to wet the Pledgers which are to be apply'd to 'em. But here are two particular and specifick Medicines to mollifie a Cancer.

Take Saccharum Saturni, Camphire, and Soot; let 'em be incorporated with the Juice of House-Leek and Plantain, in a Leaden-Mortar; then make a Liniment thereof, and cover the Part affected as lightly as is possible to be done, as with a simple Canvass-Cloth, or a Sheet of Cap-Paper: Or else, {168}

Take the destill'd Water of rotten Apples, and mingle it with the Extract of the Roots of round Birth-Wort made in Spirit of Wine; reserving this Liquor to wash the Part, and to make Injections.

* * * * *

CHAP. VIII.

Of Venereal Diseases.

Of the Chaude-pisse or Gonorrhea.

The Signs of this Disease are a painful Distention of the Penis or Yard, and a scalding Pain in making Water, the Urine being pale, whitish, and full of Filaments or little Threads: Sometimes the Testicles are swell'd as well as the

Glans and Prutrium; and sometimes there is a Flux of a kind of Matter yellowish, Greenish, &c.

If there be a great Inflammation in the Yard, endeavours must be us'd to allay it by letting Blood; and afterward the Patient may take a cooling and diuretick Diet-Drink, as also Emulsions made with cold Seeds in Whey. A very good Decoction may be prepar'd in all places, and without any trouble, by putting a Dram of Sal Prunella into every Quart of Water, whereof the Patient is to drink as often as he can: This Decoction is very cooling and diuretick; and the use of it ought to be continu'd till the Inflammation be asswag'd. Then some gentle {169} Purges are to be prescrib'd in the beginning; such as an Ounce of Cassia, and as much Manna, infus'd in two Glasses of Whey, which are to be taken one or two Hours one after another.

Afterward the Patient must be often purg'd with twelve Grains of Scammony, and fifteen Grains of Mercurius Dulcis; and these Purgations must be continu'd, till it appears that the Fluxes are neither yellowish nor greenish, nor of any other bad Colour. When they are become White, and grown Thready, they may be stopt with Astringents: Amber and dry'd Bones beaten to Powder, eighteen Grains of each, with one Grain of Laudanum, the Composition being taken in Conserve of Roses, are very good for this Purpose. Crocus Martis Astringens, or else its Extract, taken from half a Dram to a whole Dram, in like manner performs the same Operation. As soon as the Gonorrhea is stopt, to be certain of a perfect Cure, a Dram of the Mercurial Panacea is to be taken, from fifteen to twenty Grains at a time, in Conserve of Roses. In the mean while, if a small Salivation shou'd happen, it must be let alone for the present, since it may be stopt at pleasure by the Purgations. When it is requisite to restrain the Gonorrhea, Mercury must not be given any longer, in regard that it is a Dissolvent, which is only good when the Glandules of the Groin or Testicles are swell'd, or else when it is expedient to set the Chaude-pisse a running, after it hath been too suddenly stopt. At the same time that the Astringents are taken with the Mouth, {170} Injections also are to be made into the Yard; such as are prepar'd with Lapis Medicamentosus, of which one Dram is put into eight Ounces of Plantane-Water. All Astringents that are not Causticks, are proper for the Syringe.

Of Shankers.

They are round Ulcers, and hollow in the middle, which appear upon the Glans and the Prutrium. To cure 'em, they must be touch'd with the Lapis Infernalis, and brought to Suppuration by the means of red Precipitate mixt with the Ointment of Andreas Crucius. Oleum Mercurii laid on a Pledget or Bolster, is very efficacious to open Skankers, and consume their Flesh. The Patient must be well purg'd with Mercurius Dulcis and Scammony, taking twelve or fifteen Grains of each in Conserve of Roses; and after these Purgations are sufficiently reiterated, he may take the Mercurial Panacea's. It is an excellent Remedy for all sorts of Pocky Distempers not yet consummated, or arriv'd at the greatest height of Malignity.

Of Bubo's.

Bubo's are gross Tumours or Abcesses that arise in the Groin, the perfect Maturity of which is not to be waited for in order to open 'em; because it is to be fear'd lest the corrupt Matter remaining therein too long, might be convey'd into the Blood by the Circulation, and so produce the grand Pox: Therefore it is {171} necessary to open 'em betimes with a Lancet, or else with a Train of potential Cauteries, if they are too hard. They ought to be Suppurated for a considerable time: The Patient must be well purg'd with Scammony and Mercurius Dulcis: He must also take the Mercurial Panacea's.

Of the Pox.

This loathsome Disease begins sometimes with a virulent Gonorrhea, and a weariness or faintness at the same time seizeth on all the Members of the Body: It is usually accompany'd with Salivation and the Head-ach, which grows more violent at Night: Pricking Pains are also felt in the Arms and Legs, the Palate of the Mouth being sometimes ulcerated. If it be an inveterate Pox, the Bones are corrupted, and Exostoses happen therein; divers Spots with dry, round and red Pustules appear in the Skin; and the Cartilages or Gristles of the Nose are sometimes eaten up. But when this Disease is come to its greatest height of Malignity, the Hair falls off; the Gums are ulcerated; the Teeth are loose, and drop out; the whole Body is dry'd up; the Eyes are livid; the Ears tingle; the Nose become stinking; the Almonds of the Ears swell; the Uvula or Palate is down; Ulcers break out in the Privy-Parts; Bubo's arise in the Groin; as also Warts in the Glans and Prutrium; and Condyloma's in the Anus.

Indeed the Pox may be easily cur'd in the beginning; but when it hath taken deep Root {172} by a long Continuance, it is not extirpated without much difficulty, more especially if it be accompany'd with Ulcers, Caries, and Exostoses; the Person afflicted with it being of an ill Constitution, and his Voice grown hoarse.

The Spring and Summer are the proper Seasons of the Year for undertaking the Cure of this Disease: In order to which, it is necessary that the Patient begin with a regular Diet, lodging in a warm place, and taking such Aliments as yield a good Juice; as Jelly-broath made with boil'd Fowl: Let him drink Sudorifick Decoctions, prepar'd with the Wood of Guayacum, China-Root, and Sarsaparella, and let him abstain from eating any thing that is high season'd: Let him take Clysters to keep his Body open; sometimes also he may be let Blood, and purg'd with half a Dram of Jalap, and fifteen Grains of Mercurius Dulcis. The Purgations may be re-iterated as often as it shall be judg'd convenient; and then the Patient may be bath'd for nine or ten Days, every Morning and Evening; during which time he may take volatile Salt of Vipers, the Dose being from six to sixteen Grains; or else Viper's-Grease from half a Dram to a whole Dram in Conserve of Roses.

Afterward it will be necessary to proceed to Fluxing, which is caus'd by the means of Frictions with Vuguentum Mercurii, which is made of crude Mercury stirr'd about in a Mortar with Turpentine, and then the whole mingled with Hog's-Grease, one part of Mercury being usually put into two parts of Hog's-Grease. The Rubbing is begun at the Sole of the Feet, {173} by a long Continuance, it is not extirpated without ascending to the Legs, and the inside of the Thighs; but the Back-Bone must not be rubb'd at all; When the Persons are tender, or of a weak Constitution, a single Friction may be sometimes sufficient. Thus the Patient must be rubb'd at the Fire, after he hath taken a good Mess of Broath; but I would not advise it to be done with more than one or two Drams of Mercury at a time, without reckoning the Grease. Then the Patient must be dress'd with a Pair of Linnen-Drawers or Pantaloons, and laid in his Bed, where his Mouth may be lookt into from time to time, to see whether the Mercury hath taken effect; which may be easily known, by reason that his Tongue, Gums, and Palate swell and grow thick, his Head akes, his Breath is strong, his Face red, and he can scarce swallow his Spittle; or else he begins to Salivate.

If none of these Signs appear, the Rubbing must be begun again in the Morning and Evening; then if no Salivation be perceiv'd, for sometimes four or five Frictions are made successively, a little Mercurial Panacea may be taken inwardly, to promote it. During the Frictions, the Patient is to be nourish'd with Eggs, Broaths, and Gellies; he must also keep his Bed in a warm Room, and never rise till it shall be thought fit to stop the Salivation, which continues twenty or twenty five Days; or rather till it becomes Laudable; that is to say, till it be no longer stinking, nor colour'd, but clear and fluid.

If a Looseness shou'd happen during the Salivation, it wou'd cease, so that to renew it, {174} the Looseness may be stay'd with Clysters made of Milk and the Yolks of Eggs; and in case the Salivation shou'd not begin afresh, it must be excited with a slight Friction: But if it shou'd be too violent, it may be diminish'd by some gentle Purge, or with four or five Grains of Aurum Fulminans, taken in Conserve of Roses.

Three or four Pints of Rheum are commonly salivated every Day in a Bason made for that purpose, which the Patient holds in his Bed near his Mouth, so as the Spittle may run into it. But if the Fluxing shou'd not cease of it self at the time when it ought, he must be purg'd to put a stop thereto. If any Ulcers remain in his Mouth, to dry 'em up, Gargarisms are to be often us'd, which are made of Barley-Water, Honey of Roses, or luke-warm Wine.

The Warts are cur'd by binding 'em, if a Ligature be possible, or else they may be consum'd with Causticks, such as the Powder of Savine, or Aqua-fortis, by corroding the neighbouring Parts; sometimes they are cut, left to bleed for a while, and bath'd with warm Wine.

When the Patient begins to rise, he must be purg'd, his Linnen, Bed, and Chamber being chang'd; and afterward his Strength is to be recruited with good Victuals, and generous Wine. If he were too much weaken'd, let him take Cow's-Milk with Saccharum Rosatum.

If the Pox were not inveterate, the Fluxing might be excited by the Panacea alone, without any Frictions: For after the Phlebotomy, {175} Purgations, and Bathings duly administer'd; the Patient might take ten Grains of the Mercurial

Panacea in the Morning, and as many at Night; on the next Day fifteen Grains might be given, and the like quantity at Night; on the third Day twenty Grains might be given both Morning and Evening; on the fourth Day twenty five Grains in the Morning, and as many at Night; and on the fifth Day thirty Grains in the Morning, and the very same quantity in the Evening; continuing thus to augment the Dose, till the Fluxing comes in abundance; and it may be maintain'd by giving every two or every three Days twelve Grains of the Panacea. This Course must be continually follow'd till the Salivation becomes Laudable, and the Symptoms cease.

The manner of making the Mercurial Panacea.

To prepare this Panacea, it is requisite to take Mercury reviv'd from Cinnabar, because it is more pure than Mercury which is immediately dug out of the Mine. The Mercury is reviv'd with Cinnabar, after this manner: Take a Pound of artificial Cinnabar pulveriz'd, and mingled exactly with three Pounds of unslack'd Lime, in like manner beaten to Powder: Let this Mixture be put into a Retort of Stone, or Glass luted, the third part of which at least remains empty; Let it be plac'd in a reverberating Furnace; and after having fitted a Recipient fill'd with Water, let the whole be left during twenty four Hours at least; then let the Fire be {176} put under it by degrees, and at length let the Heat be very much augmented, whereupon the Mercury will run Drop by Drop into the Recipient: Let the Fire be continu'd till nothing comes forth, and the Operation will be perform'd generally in six or seven Hours: Then pour the Water out of the Recipient, and having wash'd the Mercury, to cleanse it from some small quantity of Earth that may stick thereto, let it be dry'd with Cloaths, or else with the Crum of Bread: Thus thirteen Ounces of Mercury may be drawn off from every Pound of artificial Cinnabar.

The Panacea is made of sweet Sublimate, and the later of corrosive Sublimate: To make the corrosive Sublimate, put sixteen Ounces of Mercury reviv'd from Cinnabar, into a Matrass, pour upon it eighteen Ounces of Spirit of Nitre; place the Matras upon the Sand, which must be somewhat hot, and leave it there till the Dissolution be effected: Then pour off this dissolved Liquor, which will be as clear as Water, into a Glass Vial, or into a Stone-Jug, and let its Moisture evaporate gently over the Sand-Fire, till a white Mass remains; which you may pulverize in a Glass Mortar, mingling it with sixteen Ounces of Vitriol calcin'd, and as much decrepited Salt: Put this Mixture into a

Matras, two third parts of which remain empty, and the Neck of which hath been cut in the middle of its height; then fix the Matras in the Sand, and begin to kindle a gentle Fire underneath, which may be continu'd for three Hours; afterwards let Coals be thrown upon it till the Fire burn very vehemently, and a Sublimate {177} will arise on the top of the Matras; so that the Operation may be perform'd within the space of six or seven Hours. Let the Matras be cool'd, and afterward broken; avoiding a kind of Flower or light Powder, which flyes up into the Air as soon as this Matter is remov'd; whereupon you'll find nineteen Ounces of very good corrosive Sublimate; but the red Scoria or Dross which settleth at the bottom must be cast away as unprofitable. This Sublimate being a powerful Escarotick, eats away proud Flesh, and is of singular use in cleansing old Ulcers. If half a Dram thereof be dissolv'd in a Pint of Lime-Water, it gives a yellow Tincture; and this is that which is call'd the Phagedonick-Water.

The sweet Sublimate, of which the Panacea is immediately compos'd, is made with sixteen Ounces of corrosive Sublimate, pulveriz'd in a Marble or Glass-Mortar, intermixing with it by little and little, twelve Ounces of Mercury reviv'd from Cinnabar: Let this Mixture be stirr'd about with a Wooden Pestle, till the Quick-silver become imperceptible; then put the Powder, which will be of a grey Colour, into divers Glass-Vials, or into a Matras, of which two third parts remain empty; place your Vessel on the Sand, and kindle a small Fire in the beginning, the Heat of which may be afterward encreas'd to the third Degree: Let it continue in this Condition till the Sublimate be made; and the Operation will be generally consummated {178} in four or five Hours: whereupon you may break your Vial, and throw away as useless, a little light Earth that lies at the bottom. You must also separate that which sticks to the Neck of the Vials, or of the Matras, and keep it for Ointments against the Itch; but carefully gather together the white Matter which lies in the middle, and having pulveriz'd it, cause it to be sublimated in the Vials or Matras, as before. This Matter must also be separated again (as we have already shown) and put into other Vials to be sublimated a third time. Lastly, the terrestrial parts in the bottom, and the fuliginous in the Neck of the Vials, must be, in like manner, separated, still preserving the Sublimate in the middle, which will then be very well dulcify'd, and amount to the quantity of twenty five Ounces and an half: It is an Efficacious Remedy for all sorts of Venereal Diseases; removes Obstructions, kills Worms, and purgeth gently by stool, being taken in Pills from six Grains to thirty.

Take what quantity you please of sweet Sublimate, reduce it to Powder in a Marble or Glass-Mortar, and put it into a Matras, three quarters whereof remain empty, and of which you have cut off the Neck in {179} the middle of its Height: Then place this Matras in a Furnace or Balneum of Sand, and make a little Fire underneath for an Hour, to give a gentle Heat to the Matter, which may be augmented by little and little to the third degree: Let it continue in this state about five Hours, and the Matter will be sublimated within that space of time. Then let the Vessel cool, and break it, throwing away as unprofitable a little light sort of Earth, of a reddish Colour, which is found at the bottom, and separating all the Sublimate from the Glass. Afterward pulverize it a second time, and let it be sublimated in a Matras, as before: Thus the Sublimations must be reiterated seven several times, changing the Matrasses every time, and casting away the light Earth. Then having reduc'd your Sublimate to a very fine impalpable Powder, by grinding it upon a Porphyry or Marble Stone, put it into a Glass Cucurbite or Gourd, pour into it alkaliz'd Spirit of Wine to the height of four Fingers; cover the Cucurbite with its Head, and leave the Matter in Infusion during fifteen Days, stirring it about from time to time with an Ivory Spatula. Afterward set your Cucurbite in Balneo Mari? or in a Vaporous Bath, make fit a Recipient to the Mouth of the Alembick; lute the Joints exactly with a moistened Bladder, and cause all the Spirit of Wine to be destill'd with a moderate Fire: Let the Vessels be cool'd, and unluted, andwill appear at the bottom of the Cucurbite. If it be not {180} already dry enough, you may dry it up with a gentle Fire in the Sand, stirring it with an Ivory or Wooden Spatula in the Cucurbite it self till it be reduc'd to Powder. It may be kept for use in a Glass-Vessel, as a Remedy of very great Efficacy for all sorts of Venereal Diseases, as also for Obstructions, the Scurvy, Scrophula or Kings-Evil, Tettar, Scab, Scurf, Worms, Ascarides, inveterate Ulcers, &c. The Dose is from six Grains to two Scruples, in Conserve of Roses.

* * * * *

{181}

A

TREATISE

OF THE

DISEASES

OF THE

BONES.

* * * * *

CHAP. I.

Of the Dislocation of the Bones.

What are the Diseases incident to the Bones?

They are five in number, viz. Dislocation, Fracture, Caries or Ulcer, Exostosis, and Nodus.

What is a Dislocation or Luxation?

It is the starting of the Head of one Bone out of the Cavity of another, with an {182} Interdiction of the proper Motion of the Part: Or else it is the disjointing of two Bones united together for the Motion of a Part.

How many causes are there of Dislocation in general?

Two, that is to say, one violent, and the other gentle; thus the Dislocation is made violently in Falls, Strains, Knocks, and Blows; but it is done gently and slowly in Defluctions of Rheum; as also by an insensible gathering together of Humours between the Joints, and upon the Ligaments, the Relaxation or loosening of which gives occasion afterward to the Head of the Bone to go out of its place; whence this Consequence may well be drawn, viz. that a violent Dislocation usually depends upon an external Cause, and a gentle Dislocation upon an internal.

After how many manners doth a Dislocation happen?

Two several Ways; viz. the first is called compleat, total, and perfect; and the second incompleat, partial, and imperfect: But both may happen before, behind, on the inside, and without; and may also be simple or complicated.

What are the signs of a perfect, total, and compleat Dislocation?

It is when a hard Tumour or Swelling is perceiv'd near a Hole in the place of the Joint, great pain being felt in the Part, and the Motion of it abolish'd.

What are the signs of an imperfect, partial, and incompleat Dislocation? {183}

It is when the Motion is streighten'd, and weaker than ordinary, so that some Pain is felt in the Joynt, and a Deformity may be discern'd therein, by comparing the hurt Part with the opposite which is found: This Dislocation is otherwise call'd a Sprain, when it proceeds from an external Cause; or else it is termed a Relaxation, when it happens by an internal.

What is a simple, and what is a complicated Dislocation or Luxation?

The Dislocation is properly simple, when it hath no concomitant Accidents; and it is complicated when accompany'd with some ill Symptoms or Accidents, such as Swellings, Inflammations, Wounds, Fractures, &c.

What are the means proper to be us'd in a simple Dislocation?

A speedy and simple reducing thereof, which is perform'd by stretching out the dislocated or luxated Member, and thrusting back the Head of the Bone into its natural place. Afterward the Joynt must be strengthen'd with a Fomentation made with Provence Roses, the Leaves of Wormwood, Rosemary, Camomile, St. John's-Wort, and Oak-Moss boil'd in the Lees of Wine and Forge-Water, keeping the Part well bound up, and sustain'd in a convenient situation. But if any ill Consequence is to be fear'd, apply Emplastrum Oxycroceum, or Diapalma dissolv'd in Wine.

What is to be done in a complicated Dislocation? {184}

The Accidents must be first remov'd, and then the Bone may be set, which is impossible to be done otherwise; it being dangerous even to make an Attempt before, by reason of the too great Violence with which it is effected, and which would infallibly produce a Convulsion or a Gangrene.

If the Dislocation be accompany'd with a Wound, must the Wound be cur'd before any Endeavours are us'd to reduce it?

No, but the Symptoms of the Wound, which hinder the Operation, must be taken away, as the Swelling, Inflammation, and others of the like Nature; and then it may be reduc'd, and the Wound may be dress'd according to the usual Method.

If the Dislocation be complicated with the Fracture, what is to be done then?

It is necessary to begin with reducing of the Dislocation, and afterward to perform that of the Fracture, by reason of the Extension which must be made to reduce the Dislocation, which would absolutely hinder the Setling of the Fracture.

How is the Inflammation and Swelling to be asswag'd?

With Linnen Cloaths dipt in Brandy and common Water, which must be often renew'd; or else with the Tops of Wormwood and Camomile, with Sage and Rosemary boil'd in the Lees of Wine, wherein the Bolsters and Bands are to be steep'd. But all Repercussives and Astringents must be avoided.

How doth it appear that the Reduction is well perform'd? {185}

By the Re-establishment of the Part in its natural State; by its being free from Pain; by its regular Motion; and by its conformity to the opposite Part which is found.

What Dislocations of Parts are most difficult to be reduc'd?

They are those of the Thighs with the Huckle-Bones, which are almost never perfectly set; that of the first Vertebra's is extremely difficult to be reduc'd; and those of the Lower-Jaw and Soles of the Feet are mortal.

The reducing of Dislocations is perform'd with greater facility in Infants than in Persons advanc'd in Years; but it becomes most difficult when it is deferr'd for many Days, by reason of the overflowing of the Lympha and nutritious Juice.

If an Inflammation shou'd happen before the Member is reduc'd, nothing can be done till it be allay'd, as we have already intimated; but to prevent and mitigate it, the dislocated Joynt, and the neighbouring Parts, may be bath'd with luke-warm Wine, in which hath been boil'd the Tops of St. John's-Wort, Camomile, Rosemary, Stoecas Arabica, and other Ingredients of the like Nature; the Bands must be also steept in the same Liquor.

If an Oedematous Tumour arise in the luxated Member after the Joint hath been set, it is requisite to take internal Sudorificks, and to apply Liniments made with the destill'd Oil of Tartar, and of Human Bones, which may be rectify'd with burnt Hart's Horn, or some other part of Animals, to take away its stink: Or else take yellow-Wax, and very white Rosin, {186} melt the whole Mass, and put into it white Amber and Gum Elemi, a sufficient quantity of each to make a Composition to be incorporated with Balsam of Peru; a Plaister of which may be prepar'd, and apply'd to the dislocated Member; but the Plaister must not be laid a cross, lest it shou'd contract the Part too much. The whole Member may be also anointed with Oil of St. John's-Wort, or with the destill'd Oil of Turpentine; or rather with a simple Decoction of Nervous Plants in Wine.

If the Bone be put out of its place by a coagulated sort of Matter like Mortar or Plaister, Resolutives and Attenuants are to be us'd, such as the volatile Spirit of Tartar prepar'd with the Lees of Wine, volatile Spirit of Tartar destill'd with Nitre in a Retort with a long Neck, or Spirit of Tartar prepar'd by Fermentation with Tartar, and its proper Alkali: This last is the best of all, and the use thereof ought to be continu'd. The volatile Salt of Human Bones is also very efficacious; but it is necessary to begin first with the taking of Laxative and Sudorifick Medicines, appropriated according to the respective Circumstances. The Spirit of Earth-Worms may be also apply'd outwardly, which is made by Fermentation, and may be often laid on the Part either alone, or with the Spirit of Sal Ammoniack.

If a dislocated Bone be not set in good time, a Coagulum or kind of curdled Substance is form'd in the Cavity, which hinders the reducing of it to its place; but this Coagulum may be dissolv'd with the following Medicament, before you attempt to set the Bone. Take one {187} part of the destill'd Oil of Human Bones, two parts of foetid Oil of Tartar; mingle the whole, and add quick Lime to be destill'd in a Retort: Let the Parts be fomented with this Oil.

If the Dislocation happen'd by the Relaxation of the Ligaments, recourse may be had to universal Sudorificks taken inwardly; as also to such Medicines as are full of an unctuous and volatile Salt, particularly Aromatick Oils, and Spirit of Sal Ammoniack. In the mean while Aromaticks, Resolutives, and moderate Astringents may be apply'd outwardly.

* * * * *

CHAP. II.

Of the Fractures of Bones.

What is the Fracture of a Bone?

It is the Division of the Continuity of its Parts.

After how many different manners may a Bone be broken?

Three several ways, viz. cross-wise, side-wise, in its length, and perhaps in Shatters or Splinters.

By what means may a Bone be fractured?

It may happen to be done by three sorts of Instruments, viz. such as are fit for bruising, cutting, or wresting; that is to say, a Bone may be divided in the Continuity of its proper Parts, by Contusion, Incision, or Contorsion.

How is the Fracture of a Bone discover'd? {188}

Divers ways, viz. by the ill Disposition of the Part, which becomes shorter; by its want of Motion; by its flexibility or pliantness elsewhere than in its

Articulations; by the unevenness that may be perceiv'd in its Continuity; by the cracking which is heard; sometimes also by the shooting forth of one of its ends thro' the Flesh which it hath open'd; and lastly by a Comparison made thereof with the sound Part on the other side, as that of the Right Arm with the Left.

What kind of Fracture is most difficult to be discern'd?

It is that which happens in the length of the Bone, commonly call'd a Cleft or Fissure, which gives occasion to very great Symptoms when it is unknown: But it may be found out by the Pain and Swelling felt at the bottom of the Cleft in touching it; besides the Conjectures which may be made from the Relation of the Person who hath had a Fall, and might have heard the cracking of the Bone.

What sort of Fracture is most difficult to be cur'd?

The shattering or splitting of a Bone in Pieces, by reason of the great Number of Splints which daily cause new Pains and Suppurations.

What is a simple and what is a complicated Fracture?

The simple Fracture is that whereby the Bone is broken, without any other Accident; and the complicated Fracture is that which is follow'd by some Accident; as that in which there is a splitting of the Bone in pieces, or {189} where the Bone is broken in two several places, or else when the Fracture is accompany'd with a Luxation, a Wound, an Inflammation, or other Circumstances of the like Nature.

Are old Men or Children most subject to these Fractures of the Bones?

Old Men, because their Bones are drier; whereas those of Infants are almost Cartilaginous, and yield or give way to the violence offer'd to 'em; from whence proceed the sinkings and hollowness that happen in their Skulls, especially in the Mould of their Heads, or elsewhere; for which a Remedy is found out by the means of Plaisters, Splints, and Bandages, fitted to the shape of the Parts. It is also on the same Account that Bones are more easily broken in the Winter than in the Summer.

In what Parts are the Fractures of Bones most dangerous?

They are those that happen in the Skull and Joints; in the former by reason of the Brain; and in the latter in regard of the Nervous Parts.

What Course is to be taken by a Surgeon who is sent for to cure a Fracture?

He ought to do three things, that is to say, at first he must incessantly endeavour to reduce it, to the end that Nature may re-unite the Parts with greater Facility, and that its Extremities may be brought together again with less trouble, before a Swelling, Inflammation, or Gangrene happen in the Part. Afterward he is to use means to retain the Parts in their proper Figure, and {190} natural Situation, and to prevent all sorts of Accidents.

How is the setting of a broken Bone to be perform'd?

When the Fracture is Cross-wise, it must be reduc'd by Extension and contra-Extension; and when it is in length, the Coaptation or bringing together again of the Sides, is only necessary.

What is to be done in a Fracture complicated with a Wound?

The Operator must first reduce it, and then administer the other Helps, as in a simple Fracture.

How may it be known that the reducing of the Fracture is well perform'd?

When the Pain ceaseth; when the Part hath resum'd its natural Shape; when no Unevenness is any longer perceiv'd therein; and when it is conformable to the sound Part on the other side.

What are the Signs which shew that the Splints remain in the Fracture after it hath been reduc'd?

They are the secret and continual Workings of the Fibres, or twitchings, that are felt by Intervals in the Part, with great Pains, which are the Indications of an Abcess arising therein; and when a Wound is join'd to the Fracture, the

Lips of it are puff'd up, and become more soft and pale, the purulent Matter abounding also more than ordinary.

When the Splints appear, must they be drawn out by force? {191}

By no means; for great care ought to be taken to avoid all manner of violent Operations; it being requisite to wait for their going out with the purulent Matter; or at most to facilitate their Passage by the use of Injections of the Tincture of Myrrh and Aloes; by the application of Emplastrum Andre?Crucii, and by the help of the Forceps.

How is a simple Fracture to be dress'd, after it hath been reduc'd?

The Parts are to be strengthen'd and consolidated with Liniments of Oleum Lumbricorum, or of Oil of St. John's-Wort mingled with Wine, Brandy, or Aqua-Vit? with Fomentations of Red Roses, Rosemary, and St. John's-Wort boil'd in Wine; and with Emplastrum contra Rupturam, or de Betonica, carefully wrapping up the broken Member, but after such a manner that the two Extremities may not cross one another; and that a small Space may remain open between both. Afterward the Splints and Bands are to be apply'd, taking care to avoid binding 'em too hard, and to take 'em off every three Days, in order to refit 'em, to abate troublesome Itchings, and to give Air to the Part; by these means preventing the Gangrene, which might happen by the Suffocation of the natural Heat. If the Thighs or Legs are broken, Scarves are to be us'd to support and stay 'em in the Bed.

What space of time may there be allow'd for curing the Fracture of a Bone?

The Cure will take up more or less time, according to the variety of the Parts, or the different thickness of the Bones: Thus to form {192} the Callus of the broken Jaw-Bone, twenty Days may well be allotted; for that of the Clavicle, or that of the Shoulder-Bone, twenty four; for that of the Bones of the Elbow, thirty; for that of the Arm-Bone, forty; for that of the Wrist-Bone, and those of the Fingers, twenty; for that of the Ribs, twenty; for that of the Thigh-Bone, fifty; for that of the Leg-Bone, forty; for that of the Bones of the Tarsus and Toes, twenty.

What ought to be done in particular to promote the formation of the Callus?

The fractur'd Part must be rubb'd with Oleum Lumbricorum and Spirit of Wine heated and mingled together: The Decoctions of Agrimony, Sayine, and Saxifrage are also to be us'd, and the Lapis Osteocolla is a Specifick: It is usually given in great Comphrey-Water, or in a Decoction of Perewinkle made with Wine, and is often re-iterated.

* * * * *

CHAP. III.

Of the particular Fractures of the Skull.

What is a Fracture of the Cranium or Skull?

It is a Wound of the Head complicated with a Fracture of the Skull-Bone.

After how many manners may the Skull be fractur'd? {193}

Three several ways, viz. by Contusion, by Incision, and by Puncture.

What is the most dangerous of these Fractures?

It is that which happens by Contusion; because the Concussion and Commotion is greater.

Do all the Fractures of the Skull require the use of the Trepan?

No, the Fractures must be deep which stand in need of the help of such an Instrument; for those that are superficial may be cur'd by a simple Exfoliation.

What is that deep Fracture, wherein the use of the Trepan is absolutely necessary?

It is that which is made in the two Tables of the Skull, penetrating to the Meninges of the Brain; upon which at that time the Blood is diffus'd, and must be taken away by the Operation of the Trepan.

How may it be discover'd that the two Tables of the Skull are broken?

By the Eyes, and by Ratiocination.

Are not the Eyes sufficient alone, and are they not more certain than Ratiocination?

Yes; but forasmuch as things are not always seen, there is often a necessity of making use of rational Deductions to find out that which the Eyes cannot discern.

When doth it happen that the Eyes alone discover the Fracture?

When the Wound is large and wide, so that it may be immediately view'd.

When doth it happen that Ratiocination supplies the defect of the Eyes? {194}

When the Wound is so small that the Bone cannot be seen, and nothing appears but the Accidents.

What are the Accidents or Signs of the Fracture of the Skull?

They are a dimmness of the Sight, and loss of the Understanding, which happen at the very Moment when the Fall or Blow is receiv'd; with the Phlegmatick Vomittings that follow soon after: These Signs are call'd Univocal. And there are others that bear the Name of Equivocal, and which confirm the former; as a Flux of Blood thro' the Nose, Eyes, and Ears, redness of the Eyes, heaviness of the Head, and puffing up of the Face; as also afterward Drowsiness, Shivering of the whole Body, Fever, Deliriums, Convulsions, &c.

Must all these Signs appear before a Determination can be made of the necessity of using the Trepan?

No, it is sufficient to have the Univocal Signs to make a Crucial Incision in the place of the Wound, and to lay bare the Bone, in order to observe the Fracture, which sometimes is so fine, that the Operator is oblig'd to make use of Ink, which insinuates it self into the Cleft, and of a particular Instrument, with which the black Line that hath penetrated to the bottom, cannot be rubb'd out; whereas it may be easily defac'd when the Fracture is only superficial.

How long time is commonly spent before the appearing of the Accidents?

In the Summer Season they appear in three or four Days, and at the latest in seven; in Winter {195} they are slower, and sometimes do not happen till the fourteenth Day: But at the end of this term, it may be affirm'd that the Trepan is often unprofitable.

What is requisite to be done in a doubtful Occasion; Must the Trepan be apply'd or omitted?

The Surgeon is to have recourse to his own conscientious Discretion, which ought to serve as a Guide, and requires that we should always act according to the known Rules of Art; insomuch that after having well consider'd the Accidents, with all the Circumstances of the Wound, if there be no good grounds for the undertaking of the Operation, it is expedient to desist, and in this case to have deference to the Advice of other able Surgeons of the same Society, rather than to rely too much upon his own Judgment, to the end that he may be always secure from all manner of Blame.

Is the Trepan apply'd upon the Fracture?

No; but on one side of it, and always in a firm place.

What Course is to be taken when a Fracture is found in a Suture?

A double Trepan is to be made, and apply'd on each side of the Suture, by reason of the overflowing of the Blood, which may happen therein.

What Method ought to be observ'd in the curing of the Wounds of the Head, and Fractures of the Skull?

In simple Wounds of the Head, it is necessary only to make use of Balsams, and to lay over 'em Emplastrum de Betonica. When there is a Contusion either in the {196} Pericranium, or in the Skull, the Wound must be kept open till after the Suppuration or Exfoliation.

When there is only a Bunch without any Wound or Accident, it must speedily be dissolv'd with Plaister or Mortar, Chimney-Soot, Oil of Olives, and Wine, laid upon the Part between two Linnen-Rags; or else with Soot, Spirit of Wine, and Oil of St. John's-Wort, wherein the Bolsters are soakt, to be in like manner apply'd with a Band.

Wounds of the Head accompany'd with a Fracture, absolutely require the application of the Trepan, wherein it is requisite to make use of Oil of Turpentine to be dropt upon the Membrane of the Brain; or else Spirit of Wine mingled with Oil of Almonds, and not with the Oil or Syrrup of Roses; and to endeavour to cause a plentiful outward Suppuration.

Besides, it must not be neglected to enjoyn the wounded Person to be let Blood both before and after the Operation, if he hath a Fever or a Plethory; and more especially it is to be remember'd to cause his Body to be kept open at least every other Day, with Clysters, obliging him to keep a good Diet, and to avoid all violent Agitations both of Body and Mind, abstaining from eating Flesh till the Fourteenth Day. All manner of Venery and Conjugal Embraces, which prove fatal at this time, are to be prohibited during forty Days, to be counted from the Day of the Operation; as they are also in all other considerable Wounds.

* * * * *

{197}

CHAP. IV.

Of the Caries or Ulcer of the Bones, Exostosis, and Nodus.

What is Caries?

It is the Putrifaction of the Substance of the Bone, or else its Ulcer or Gangrene.

Whence doth the Caries of the Bone derive its Original?

It proceeds from an internal and external Cause; the former being that which hath been produc'd at first in the Substance of the Bone; and the other that which takes its Rise from an inveterate Ulcer in the Flesh, which hath communicated its Malignity to the Substance of the Bone, and by that means corrupted it.

How is the Caries known which proceeds from an inward Cause?

By the continual and violent Pains which are felt before, and continue for a long time without diminution; as also afterward by the alteration of the Flesh that covers the Bone, and which becomes soft, spongy, and livid.

By what means is a Caries that derives its Origine from an outward Cause, discover'd?

By the quality of the purulent Matter that issueth out of the Ulcer in the Flesh, which is blackish, Unctuous, and extremely stinking; as also by the help of the Probe, that discovereth {198} asperity or roughness in the Bone when it is laid bare.

What Means are to be us'd in order to cure a Caries proceeding from an external Cause?

The Powder of Flower-de-luce may be us'd, and it is sufficient for that purpose, when the Caries is superficial; but it is necessary to take Oleum Guyaci, and to soak Bolsters therein, to be laid upon the Ulcer when it is deep; or else Aqua-Vit?or Brandy, in which have been infus'd the Roots of Flower-de-luce, Cinnamon, and Cloves. Lastly, the actual Cautery, which is Fire, must be apply'd thereto.

What is to be done when the Caries proceeds from an internal Cause?

The Flesh must be open'd to give Passage to the Sanies that runs out of the ulcerated Bone, to the end that Exfoliation may be procur'd; and if the Ulcer hath not as yet laid open the Bone on the outside, the Trepan ought to be apply'd; but the Ulcer or Caries must be afterward handled, as we have even now declar'd.

What is Exostosis?

It is the Swelling of a Bone made by the settling of a corrupt Humour in its proper Substance.

What is Nodus?

It is a kind of gummy and wavering Tumour, which is form'd by the settling of a gross Humour between the Bone and the Periosteum.

Are Exostoses and Nodus's suppurable Tumours?

Yes, because they sometimes produce Ulcers and Gangrenes in the Bone, which are call'd {199} Caries, proceeding from an internal Cause; nevertheless they are generally dissolv'd by Frictions with Unguentum Griseum, or by the application of Plaisters of Tobacco, or Emplastrum de Vigo quadruplicato Mercurio; taking also to the same purpose internal Diaphoretick and Sudorifick Medicines, with convenient Purgatives.

* * * * *

CHAP. V.

Of Cauteries, Vesicatories, Setons, Cupping-Glasses, and Leeches.

What is a Vesicatory?

The Name of Vesicatory may be attributed to every thing that is capable of raising Bladders or Blisters in the Skin; nevertheless in Surgery, by a Vesicatory is understood a Medicament prepar'd with Cantharides or Spanish Flies dried, which are beaten to Powder, and mingled with Turpentine, Plaisters, Leaven, and other Ingredients.

In what places, and after what manner are Vesicatories usually apply'd?

They are apply'd every where, accordingly as there is occasion to draw out or discharge some Humour from a Part: In Defluxions of Rheum upon the

Eyes or Teeth, they are laid on the Neck and Temples; in Apoplexies, behind the Ears; and so of the rest, observing always to make Frictions on the places where the {200} Application is to be made, to the end that the Vesicatory may sooner take effect.

How long time must the Vesicatory continue on the Part?

The Blisters are generally rais'd by 'em within the space of five or six Hours; yet this Operation depends more or less upon the fineness of the Skin; and when the Bladders or Blisters appear, it is requisite to deferr the openning of 'em for some time, to the end that Nature may have an Opportunity to introduce a new Scarf-Skin, by which means the Pain may be avoided that would be felt, if the Skin were too much expos'd to the Air.

What is a Cautery?

It is a Composition made of many Ingredients, which corrode, burn, and make an Escar on the Part to which they are apply'd.

How many sorts of Cauteries are there in general?

There are two kinds, viz. the Actual and the Potential; the former are those that have an immediate Operation; as Fire, or a red-hot Iron; and the others are those that produce the same Effect, but in a longer space of time; such are the ordinary Cauteries compos'd of Caustick Medicaments.

Which are the most safe, the Actual or the Potential Cauteries?

A distinction is to be made herein; for Actual Cauteries are safest in the Operation, because they may be apply'd wheresoever one shall think fit, as also for as long a time, or for any purpose: Whereas the Potential cannot be {201} guided after the same manner. But in Hemorrhages the Potential Cauteries are most eligible, by reason that the Escar produc'd by 'em not being so speedily form'd, the Vessels are better clos'd, and they are not so subject to open again when it falls off; as it often happens in the Fall of an Escar made by Fire.

In what places are Cauteries usually apply'd?

In all places where an Attraction is to be made, or an Intemperature to be corrected, or a Flux of Humours to be stopt, by inducing an Escar on the Part: However they are commonly laid upon the Nape of the Neck, between the first and second Vertebra; on the outward Part of the Arm in a small Hole between the Muscle Deltoides and the Biceps; above the Thigh, between the Muscle Sartor, and the Vastus Internus; and on the inside of the Knee, below the Flexors of the Leg; observing every where that the Cautery be plac'd near the great Vessels, to the end that it may draw out and cleanse more abundantly.

What is the Composition of the Potential Cauteries?

They may be made with quick Lime, Soap, and Chimney-Soot; or else take an Ounce of Sal Ammoniack, two Ounces of burnt Roman Vitriol, three Ounces of quick Lime, and as many of calcin'd Tartar; mingle the whole Mass together in a Lixivium of Bean-Cod Ashes, and cause it to evaporate gently to a Consistence: Let this Paste be kept for use in a dry place, and in a well-stopt Vessel. Or else the Silver-Cautery, or Lapis Infernalis may be prepar'd after the following manner: {202}

Take what quantity you please of Silver, let it be dissolv'd with thrice as much Spirit of Nitre in a Vial, and set the Vial upon the Sand-Fire, to the end that two third parts of its Moisture may evaporate: Then pour the rest scalding-hot into a good Crucible, plac'd over a gentle Fire, and the Ebullition being made, the heat of the Fire must be augmented, till the Matter sink to the bottom, which will become as it were an Oil: Afterward pour it into a somewhat thick and hot Mould, and it will coagulate, so as to be fit for Use, if it be kept in a well-stopt Vial. This Cautery is the best; and an Ounce of Silver will yield one Ounce and five Drams of Lapis Infernalis.

What is a Seton?

It is a String of Silk, Thread, or Cotton, threaded thro' a kind of Pack-Needle, with which the Skin of a Part is to be pierc'd thro', to make an Ulcer therein, that hath almost the same effect as a Cautery.

What is most remarkable in the Application of a Seton?

It ought to be observ'd, that the String must be dipt in Oil of Roses, and that one end of it must always be kept longer than the other, to facilitate the running of the Humours.

In what Parts is the Seton to be apply'd?

The Nape of the Neck is the usual place of its Application, altho' it may be made in any part of the Body where it is necessary. It sometimes happens that a Surgeon is oblig'd to use a kind of Seton in such Wounds made with a Sword, or by Gun-shot, as pass quite {203} thro' from one side to the other; then the String or Skain must be dipt in convenient Ointments or Medicinal Compositions; and as often as the Dressings are taken away, it will be requisite to cut off the Part soakt in the Purulent Matter, which must be taken out of the Ulcer.

What is a Cupping-Glass?

It is a Vessel or kind of Vial, made with Glass, the bottom whereof is somewhat broader than the top, which is apply'd to the Skin to cause an Attraction. There are two sorts of these Cupping-Glasses, viz, the Dry, and the Wet; the former are those that are laid upon the Skin without opening it; and the latter those that are apply'd with Scarification.

In what Diseases are Cupping-Glasses us'd?

In all kinds where it is necessary to make any Attraction; but more especially in Apoplexies, Vapours in Women, Palsies, and other Distempers of the like Nature. But the Applications of Cupping-Glasses are altogether different; for in Apoplexes they are generally set upon the Shoulders or upon the Coccyx; in Vapours upon the inside of the Thighs; and in Palsies upon the Paralytick Part it self.

What is a Leech?

It is an Animal like a little Worm which sucks the Blood, and is commonly apply'd to Children and weak Persons, to serve instead of Phlebotomy: Leeches are also us'd for the discharging of a Defluxion of Humours in any

Part; as also in the Hemorrhoidal Veins when they are too full; in the Varices and in several parts of the Face. {204}

What choice ought to be made of Leeches?

It is requisite to take those that have their Backs greenish, and their Bellies red; as also to seek for 'em in a clear running Stream, and to cast away those that are black and hairy.

* * * * *

CHAP. VI.

Of Phlebotomy.

What is Phlebotomy?

It is an evacuation of Blood procur'd by the artificial Incision of a Vein or Artery, with a design to restore Health.

Which are the Vessels that are open'd in Phlebotomy or Blood-letting?

They are in general all the Veins and Arteries of the Body, nevertheless some of 'em are more especially appropriated to this Operation; as the Vena Preparata in the Forehead; the Ranul?under the Tongue; the Jugular Veins and Arteries in the Neck; the Temporal Arteries in the Temples; the Cephalick, Median, and Basilick Veins in the inside of the Elbow; the Salvatella between the Ring-Finger and the Little-Finger; the Poplit in the Ham; the Saphena in the internal Malleolus or Ankle; and the Ischiatica in the external.

What are the Conditions requisite in the due performing of the Operation of Phlebotomy?

They are these, viz. to make choice of a proper Vessel; not to open any at all Adventures; not to let Blood without necessity, nor {205} without the Advice of a Physician; whose Office it is to determine the Seasons or Times convenient for that purpose; as that of Intermission in an Intermitting Fever; that of Cooling in the Summer; and that of Noon-tide in the Winter; and lastly, to take away different quantities of Blood; for in the Heat of Summer they ought to be lesser, and greater in the Winter.

What are the Accidents of Phlebotomy?

They are an Impostume, a Rhombus, an Echymosis, an Aneurism, Lipothymy, Swooning, and a Convulsion.

What is a Rhombus?

It is a small Tumour of the Blood which happens in the place where the Operation is perform'd either by making the Orifice too small, or larger than the Capaciousness of the Vessel will admit. The Rhombus is cur'd by laying upon it a Bolster dipt in fair Water, between the Folds of which must be put a little Salt, to dissolve and prevent the Suppuration.

How may it be perceiv'd that an Artery hath been prickt or open'd in letting Blood?

The Puncture of an Artery produceth an Aneurism; and the Opening of it causeth a Flux of Vermilion Colour'd Blood, which issueth forth in abundance, and by Leaps.

Are the Leaps which the Blood makes in running, a certain Sign that it comes from an Artery?

No, because it may so happen, that the Basilick Vein lies directly upon an Artery, the beating of which may cause the Blood of the {206} Basilica to run out leaping: Therefore these three Circumstances ought to be consider'd jointly, that is to say, the Vermilion Colour, the great quantity and the Leaps, in order to be assur'd that the Blood proceeds from an Artery.

How may it be discover'd that a Tendon hath been hurt in letting Blood?

It is known when in opening the Median Vein, the end of the Lancet hath met with some Resistance; when the Patient hath felt great Pain, and afterward when the Tendon apparently begins to be puff'd up, and the Arm to swell. A Remedy may be apply'd to this Accident thus; after having finish'd the Operation, a Bolster steep'd in Oxycratum is to be laid upon the Vessel, a proper Bandage is to be made, and the Arm must be wrapt up in a Scarf: If the Inflammation that ariseth in the Part be follow'd with Suppuration, it must be dress'd with a small Tent; and if the Suppuration be considerable, it is necessary to dilate the Wound, and to make use of Oil of Eggs and Brandy, with a good Digestive; as also to apply Emplastrum Ceratum; to make an Embrocation on the Arm with Oil of Roses; and to dip the Bolsters in Oxycratum to cover the whole Part.

Is it not to be fear'd that some Nerve may be wounded in letting Blood?

No, they lie so deep that they cannot be touch'd.

Under what Vein is the Artery of the Arm?

It is usually situated under the Basilica. {207}

What Course is proper to be taken to avoid the Puncture of an Artery in letting Blood?

It must be felt with the Hand before the Ligature is made, observing well whether it be deep or superficial; for when it lies deep, there is nothing to be fear'd; and when it is superficial, it may be easily avoided by pricking the Vein either higher or lower.

What is to be done when an Artery is open'd?

If it be well open'd, it is requisite to let the Blood run out till the Person falls into a Syncope or Swoon, by which means the Aneurism is prevented; and afterward the Blood will be more easily stopt: It remains only to make a good Bandage with many Bolsters, in the first of which is simply put a Counter or a Piece of Money; but a bit of Paper chew'd will serve much better, with Bolsters laid upon it in several Folds.

If the Arteries cause so much trouble when open'd accidentally, why are those of the Temples sometimes open'd on purpose, to asswage violent Pains in the Head?

By reason that in this place the Arteries are situated upon the Bones that press 'em behind; which very much facilitates their re-union.

Are not the Arteries of Persons advanc'd in Years more difficult to be clos'd than those of Children?

Yes. {208}

Are there not Accidents to be fear'd in letting Blood in the Foot?

Much less than in the Arm; because the Veins of the Malleoli or Ankles are not accompany'd either with Arteries or Tendons; which gave occasion to the Saying, That the Arm must be given to be let Blood only to an able Surgeon, but the Foot may be afforded to a young Practitioner.

* * * * *

{209}

A

TREATISE

OF

Chirurgical Operations.

* * * * *

CHAP. I.

Of the Operation of the Trepan.

This Operation is to be perform'd, when it is inferr'd from the Signs of which we have already given a particular Account, that some Matter is diffus'd over the Dura Mater. The Trepan must not be us'd in the Sinus Superciliares, by reason of their Cavity; nor in the Sutures, in regard of the Vessels that pass thro' 'em; nor in the Temporal Bone without great necessity, especially in that part of it which is join'd to the Parietal-Bone, lest the end of this Bone shou'd fly out of its place, since it is only laid upon the Parietal; nor in the middle of the Coronal and Occipital-Bones, by reason of an inner {210} Prominence wherein they adhere to the Dura Mater; nor in the Passage of the Lateral Sinus's that are situated on the side of the Occipital.

If the Fissure be very small, the Trepan may be apply'd upon it, altho' it is more expedient to use this Instrument on the side of the Fissure in the lower part; neither is the Trepan to be set upon the Sinkings; and if the Bones are loosen'd or separated, there needs no other trepanning than to take 'em away with the Elevatory.

The Operation must be begun with Incision, which is usually made in form of a Cross, if the Wound be remote from the Sutures, and there are no Muscles to be cut, and in the shape of the Letter T. or of the Figure 7. if it be near the Sutures, so that the Foot of the 7. or of the T. ought to be parallel to the Suture, the top of the Letter descending toward the Temples; it is also made in the middle of the Forehead. If it be sufficient to make a longitudinal Incision in the Forehead; its Wrinkles may be follow'd, and there will be less Deformity in the Scar; but it is never done Crosswise in this Part, and the Lips of the Wound are not to be cut. If an Incision be made on the Muscle Crotaphites, and on those of the back-part of the Head, it may be done in form of the Letter V. the Point of which will stand at the bottom of the Muscles; nevertheless it is more convenient to make a longitudinal Incision, by which means fewer Fibres will be cut; and it is always requisite to begin at the lower part, to avoid being hindred by the Hemorrhage. {211} The Incisions are to be made with the Incision-Knife, and that too boldly when there are no Sinkings; but if there be any, too much weight must not be laid upon 'em: Thus the Incision being finish'd, the Lips of the Skull are to be separated either with the Fingers, or some convenient Instrument; Then if there be no urgent Occasion to apply the Trepan, it may be deferr'd till the next Day, the Wound being dress'd in the mean time with Plaisters, Bolsters, Pledgets, and a large Kerchief or upper Dressing, the use of which we shall shew hereafter.

The Operation is begun with the Perforative, to make a little Hole for the fixing of the Pyramid or Pin which is in the Round; afterward the Round is to be apply'd, holding the Handle of the Trepan with the Left-hand, and turning with the other very fast in the beginning; but when the Round hath made its way, it is lifted up to remove the Pin, lest this Point shou'd hurt the Dura Mater: Thus the Round being taken off from time to time, to be cleans'd from the Filings that stick thereto, is set on again, and the Operator begins his Work of turning anew, which must be carry'd on gently when any Blood appears, to the end that the first Table of the piece of Bone which is remov'd may not fly from the second: When it comes near the Dura Mater, the Operator must proceed, in like manner, gently, searching with a Feather round about the Bone, to observe whether he still continueth his Course in the Skull. He must also often lift up the Trepan to search the Hole, to cleanse the Instrument, and to keep {212} it from growing hot. As often as the Trepan is taken off, let him search with a Feather, to see whether the Bone be cut equally; and if it be not, he must lean more on that side which is least cut. If it be necessary to make use of the Terebella, the Hole must be made in the beginning, whilst the Bone is as yet firm; and when the Piece begins to move, the Terebella is to be put very gently into its Hole, without pressing the Bone, to draw it out; or else it may be taken away with the Myrtle-Leaf, which is an Instrument made of a firm Silver-Plate somewhat crooked. When the Piece is thus remov'd, the uneven Parts that remain at the bottom of the Hole, are to be cut with the Lenticula; and if there be any Sinkings, they may be rais'd with the Elevatory. Whereupon the Dura Mater may be compress'd a little with the Lenticula, to facilitate the running out of the Blood, the Wounded Person being oblig'd to stoop with his Head downward, stopping his Nose and Mouth, and holding his Breath for a while, to cause the Matter to run out: Then the Dura Mater may be wip'd with Lint; but if any Pus or corrupt Matter lies underneath, it must be pierc'd with a Lancet wrapt up in a Tent, that it may not be perceiv'd by the Assistants. Afterward a Sindon or very fine Linnen Rag dipt in a proper Medicament, is put between the Dura Mater and the Skull; the Hole is fill'd with small Bolsters steept in convenient Medicinal Liquors; and the Wound is dress'd with Pledgets, a Plaister, and a Kerchief. {213}

But the Hole ought to be well stopt with Bolsters, because the Dura Mater is sometimes so much inflam'd, that it bursts forth; so that if any Excrescences arise therein, and go out of the Hole, having small Roots, they may be bound and cut; but if their Roots be large, they must be press'd close with little Bolsters steept in Spirituous Medicines. Here it may not be improper to observe, that the Operation of the Trepan ought to be perform'd more gently in Children than in adult Persons, in regard that their Bones are more tender, and that Oily Medicines must not be us'd, but Spirituous. The Exfoliation is made sometimes sooner, and sometimes later; but the Callus usually covers the opening of the Skull within the space of forty or fifty Days, if no ill Accident happens. In great Fractures, where there is no longer any connexion between the Bones, it is requisite to take 'em away.

Of the Bandage of the Trepan.

The proper Bandage to be us'd after the Operation of the Trepan, is the great Kerchief, which is a large Napkin folded into two parts after such a manner that the side which toucheth the Head exceeds that which doth not touch it in the breadth of four Fingers; it is apply'd to the Head in the middle, whilst a Servant holds the Dressing with his Hand: Then the two upper ends of the Napkin being brought under Chin, the Surgeon takes the two lower, and draws 'em streight by the sides, so as that side the Napkin, which is four Fingers broader {214} than the other, may be laid upon the Forehead: Afterward the two ends of the Napkin are cross'd behind the Head, and fasten'd at their Extremities with Pins, without making any Folds, that might hurt the Part; but the ends of the Napkin which fall upon the Shoulders, are rais'd up to the Head near the lesser Corner of the Eyes; and the two ends under the Chin are fasten'd with Pins, or else tied in a Knot.

* * * * *

CHAP. II.

Of the Operation of the Fistula Lachrymalis.

This Operation is perform'd when there is a Fistulous Ulcer in the great Corner of the Eye, after this manner: The Patient being plac'd in a convenient Posture, and having his sound Eye bound up, to take away the sight of the Instruments; the Operator causeth the other Eye to be kept steady with a Bolster held with an Instrument, and makes an Incision with a Lancet in form of a Crescent upon the Tumour, taking care to avoid cutting the Eye-Lid and the little Cartilage which serves as a Pulley to the great Oblique Muscle. If the Bone be putrify'd with a Caries, an Actual Cautery may be apply'd thereto, using for that purpose a small Funnel or Tube, thro' the Canal of which the Cautery is convey'd to the Bone. {215} But the Bone must not be pierc'd, for it is exfoliated entire by reason of its smallness; and so the Hole is made without any Perforation.

The Dressing and Bandage of the Fistula Lachrymalis.

The Wound is fill'd with small dry Pledgets, and cover'd with a Plaister and Bolster: The Bandage is made with an Handkerchief folded triangular-wise, the ends of which are fasten'd behind the Head. If the Flesh grows too fast, it may be consum'd with the Lapis Infernalis; and if there be occasion to dilate the Wound, to facilitate the Exfoliation, it may be done with little pieces of Spunge prepar'd, and put into it. Afterward Causticks are to be us'd, to eat away the Callous Parts, which may be mingled with Oily Medicines, to weaken their Action, taking care, nevertheless, that the Eye receive no dammage by 'em. If the Bone be corrupted, a little Euphorbium may be apply'd; or else the small Pledgets steept in the Tincture of Myrrh and Aloes; then the Ulcer may be handled as all others.

* * * * *

{216}

CHAP. III.

Of the Operation of the Cataract.

This Operation is perform'd when there is a small Body before the Apple of the Eye, which hinders the Sight from entring into it; but it is undertaken only in Blew, Green, and Pearl-colour'd Cataracts, or in those that are of the Colour of polish'd Steel; and not in Yellow, Black, or Lead-colour'd. To know whether the Cataract be fit to be couch'd, the Patient's Eye must be rubb'd; so that if the Cataract remains unmoveable, it is mature enough; but if it changeth its place, it is requisite to wait till it become more solid. The Spring and Autumn are the most proper Seasons for performing the Operation.

To this purpose the Patient being set down with his Eyes turn'd toward the Light, and having his sound Eye bound up, the Surgeon must likewise sit on a higher Seat, whilst the Patient's Head is held by a Servant; and his Eye being turn'd toward his Nose, is kept steady with a Speculum Oculi, which is a little

Iron-Instrument made like a Spoon, pierc'd in the middle, so that the Ball of the Eye may be let thro' this Hole: Then the Surgeon taking a Steel-Needle either round or flat, accordingly as he shall judge convenient, perforates the Conjunctive at the end of the Corneous Tunicle, on the side of the little Corner of the {217} Eye, and boldly thrusts his Needle into the middle of the Cataract, which he at first pusheth upward, to loosen it with the Point of the Needle; and then downward, holding it for some time with his Needle below the Apple of the Eye. If it ascend again after it is let go, it must be depress'd a second time; but the Operation is finish'd when it remains in the same place whereto it was thrust; neither is the Needle to be remov'd till this be done, and the Cataract entirely couch'd. In taking out the Needle, the Eye-Lid must be pull'd down, and press'd a little over the Eye.

The Dressing and Bandage,

Is to cause both the Patient's Eyes to be clos'd and bound up; then he must be oblig'd to keep his Bed during seven or eight Days, and some Defensative is to be laid upon the sore Eye, to hinder the Inflammation.

M. Dupr? Surgeon to the Hospital of Hotel-Dieu at Paris, a Person well vers'd in these kinds of Operations, hath observ'd, that after the same manner as Cataracts were form'd in a very little space of time in perfect Maturity; it happen'd also very often, that the Cataracts which were suppos'd to have got up again, were not the very same with those that were couch'd, but rather a new Pellicula or little Skin, which sometimes hath its Origine in the top of the Uveous Tunicle, and is caus'd only by a very considerable Relaxation of the Excretory Vessels from the Sources of the Aqueous Humour which in filtrating permits the running {218} of many heterogeneous Parts, the Encrease of which produceth a new Cataract.

Of other Operations in the Eyes.

Sometimes a sort of purulent Matter is gather'd together under the Corneous Tunicle; so that to draw it out, the Eye must be fixt in a Posture with the Speculum Oculi, and after a small Incision made therein with a fine Lancet, is to be press'd a little, to let out the Matter; but if it be too thick, it may be drawn forth by sucking gently with a small Tube or Pipe, having a little Vial in the middle, into which the Matter will fall as it is suck'd out.

Sometimes a small Tumour ariseth in the Eye, which being ty'd at its Root with a Slip-Knot, to streighten it from time to time, will at length be dissolv'd: But if the Tumour lie in the Hole of the Apple of the Eye, this Operation must not be admitted, lest the Scar shou'd hinder the Passage of the Light. Sometimes also a somewhat hard Membrane, call'd Unguis, appears in the great corner of the eye, which when it sticks thereto, may be cut off by binding it; this is done with a Needle and Thread, which is pass'd thro' the Membrane, and afterward ty'd.

If the Eye-Lids are glu'd together, a crooked Needle without a Point may be threaded, and pass'd underneath 'em; then the ends of the Thread may be drawn, to lift up the Eye-Lids, and they may be separated with a Lancet.

{219}

If the Hairs of the Eye-Lids or Eye-Brows offend the Eye, they must be pull'd out with a Pair of Tweezers or Nippers; and when any small, hard, and transparent Tumours arise in the Eye-Lids, they are to be open'd, to let out the corrupt Matter.

* * * * *

CHAP. IV.

Of the Operation of the Polypus.

This Operation is necessary, when there are any Excrescences of Flesh in the Nostrils, which, nevertheless, when they are livid, stinking, hard, painful, and sticking very close, must not be tamper'd with, because they are Cancers. But if they are whitish, red, hanging, and free from Pain, the Cure may be undertaken after this manner: Take hold of the Polypus with a Pair of Forceps, as near its Root as is possible, and turn 'em first on one side, and then on another, till it be pull'd off. If the Polypus descends into the Throat, it may be drawn thro' the Mouth with crooked Forceps; and if an Hemorrhage shou'd happen after the Operation, it may be stopt by thrusting up into the Nostrils certain Tents soakt in some Styptick Liquor; or else by Syringing with the same Liquor.

* * * * *

{220}

CHAP. V.

Of the Operation of the Hare-Lip.

This Operation is perform'd when the Upper-Lip is cleft; but if there be a great loss of Substance, it must not be undertaken; neither ought it to be practis'd upon old nor scorbutick Persons, nor upon young Children, by reason that their continual Crying wou'd hinder the re-union. But if any are desirous that it shou'd be done to these last, they are to be kept from taking any rest for a long time, to the end that they may fall a-sleep after the Operation, which is thus effected:

If the Lip sticks to the Gums, it is to be separated with an Incision-Knife, without hurting 'em; then the Hare-Lip must be cut a little about the edges with Sizzers, that it may more easily re-unite, the edges being held for that purpose with a Pair of Pincers, whilst the Servant who supports the Patient's Head, presseth his Cheeks before, to draw together the sides of the Hare-Lip: Whereupon the Operator passeth a Needle with wax'd Thread, into the two sides of the Wound, from the outside to the inside at a Thread's distance from each. But care must be had that the two Lips of the Hare-Lip be well adjusted, and very even; the Thread being twisted round the Needle by crossing it above.

{221}

The Dressing and Bandage.

After the Lips are wash'd with warm Wine, the Points of the Needles must be cut off, small Bolsters being laid under their ends; then the Wound is to be dress'd with a little Pledget cover'd with some proper Balsam, putting at the same time under the Gum a Linnen Rag steep'd in some desiccative Liquor, lest the Lip shou'd stick to the Gum, if it be necessary to keep 'em a-part. Lastly, upon the whole is to be laid an agglutinative Plaister, supported with the uniting Bandage, which is a small Band perforated in the middle; it is laid behind the Head, and afterward drawn forward, one of its ends being let into the Hole which lies upon the Sore: Then the two ends of the Band are turn'd behind the Head upon the same Folds where they are fasten'd, sticking therein a certain Number of Pins, proportionably to the length of the Wound.

The Patient must be dress'd three Days after; and it is requisite at the first time only to untwist half the Needle, loosening the middle Thread if there be three; to which purpose a Servant is to thrust the Cheeks somewhat forward. On the eighth Day the middle Needle may be taken off, if it be a young Infant; nevertheless the Needles must not be remov'd till it appears that the sides are well join'd; neither must they be left too long, because the Holes wou'd scarce be brought to close.

* * * * *

{222}

CHAP. VI.

Of the Operation of Bronchotomy.

This Operation becomes necessary, when the Inflammation that happens in the Larynx hinders Respiration, and is perform'd after this manner:

The Wind-Pipe is open'd between the third and fourth Ring, above the Muscle Cricoides, or else in the middle of the Wind-Pipe; but in separating the Muscles call'd Sternohyodei, care must be had to avoid cutting the recurrent Nerves, lest the Voice shou'd be lost; as also the Glandules nam'd Thyroides. The Space between the Rings is to be open'd with a streight Lancet, kept steady with a little Band, and a transverse Incision is to be made between 'em: Before the Lancet is taken out, a Stilet is put into the Opening, thro' which passeth a little Pipe, short, flat, and somewhat crooked at the end, which must not be thrust in too far, for fear of exciting a Cough. This Pipe hath two small Rings for the fastening of Ribbans, which are ty'd round about the Neck; and it must be left in the Wound till the Symptoms cease. Afterward it is taken away, and the Wound is dress'd, the Lips of it being drawn together again with the uniting Bandage, which hath been already describ'd.

* * * * *

{223}

CHAP. VII.

Of the Operation of the Uvula.

When the Uvula or Palate of the Mouth is swell'd so as to hinder Respiration or Swallowing, or else is fallen into a Gangrene, it may be extirpated thus: The Tongue being first depress'd with an Instrument call'd Speculum Oris, the Palate is held with a Forceps, or cut with a Pair of Sizzers; or else a Ligature may be made before it is cut; and the Mouth may be afterward gargl'd with Astringent Liquors.

* * * * *

CHAP. VIII.

Of the Operation of a Cancer in the Breast.

The Cancer at first is not so big as a Pea, being a small, hard, blackish Swelling, sometimes livid, and very troublesome by reason of its Prickings; but when it is encreas'd, the Tumour appears hard, Lead-colour'd, and livid, causing in the beginning a Pain that may be pretty well endur'd, but in the increase it grows intolerable, and the Stink is extremely noisome. When it is ready to Ulcerate, the Heat is vehement, with a pricking Pulsation; and the Veins round about are turgid, being {224} fill'd with black Blood, and extended as it were the Feet of a Crab or Crey-Fish, till Death happen. When this Tumour is not ulcerated, it is call'd an Occult Cancer; and an Apparent one when it breaks forth into an open Ulcer.

To palliate an Occult Cancer, and prevent its Ulceration, a Cataplasm or Pultis of Hemlock very fresh may be apply'd to the Part. All the kinds of Succory, the Decoction of Solanum or Night-shade; the Juices of these Plants, as also those of Scabious, Geranium or Stork-Bill, Herniaria or Rupture-Wort,

Plantain, &c. are very good in the beginning. River-Crabs pounded in a Leaden-Mortar, and their Juice beaten in a like Mortar, are an excellent Remedy; as also are Humane Excrements or Urine destill'd, and laid upon the Occult Cancer: Or else,

Take an Ounce of calcin'd Lead, two Ounces of Oil of Roses, and six Drams of Saffron; let the whole Composition be beaten in a Mortar with a Leaden Pestle, and apply'd. The Amalgama of Mercury with Saturn is likewise a very efficacious Remedy.

In the mean while the Patient may be purg'd with black Hellebore and Mercurius Dulcis, taking also inwardly from one Scruple to half a Dram of the Powder of Adders, given to drink, with half the quantity of Crab's-Eyes: But very great care must be taken to avoid the Application of Maturatives or Emollients, which wou'd certainly bring the Tumour to Ulceration. {225}

When the Cancer is already ulcerated, the Spirit of Chimney-Soot may be us'd with good Success; and the Oil of Sea-Crabs pour'd scalding hot into the Ulcer, is an excellent Remedy. But if it be judg'd expedient entirely to extirpate the Cancer, it may be done thus:

The sick Patient being laid in Bed, the Surgeon takes the Arm on the side of the Cancer, and lifts it upward and backward, to give more room to the Tumour; then having pass'd a Needle with a very strong Thread thro' the bottom of the Breast, he cuts the Thread to take away the Needle, and passeth the Needle again into the Breast, to cause the Threads to cross one another. Afterward these four ends of the Threads are ty'd together, to make a kind of Handle to take off the Tumour, which is cut quite round to the Ribs with a very sharp Rasor. The Cutting is usually begun in the lower Part to end in the Vessels near the Arm-Pit, where a small Piece of Flesh is left, to stop the Blood with greater Facility: Then having laid a Piece of Vitriol upon the Vessels, or Bolsters soakt in styptick Water; the sides of the Breast are to be press'd with the Hand, to let out the Blood and Humours; and an Actual Cautery is to be lightly apply'd thereto.

The Dressing.

The Wound is to be dress'd with Pledgets strew'd with Astringent Powders, a Plaister, a Bolster, a Napkin round the Brest, and a Scapulary to support the whole Bandage. {226}

But instead of passing Threads cross-wise, to form a Handle, with which the Breast may be taken off, it wou'd be more expedient to make use of a sort of Forceps turn'd at both ends in form of a Crescent, after such a manner that those ends may fall one upon another when the Forceps are shut. Thus the Surgeon may lay hold on the Breast with these Forceps, and draw it off, after having cut it at one single Stroak with a very flat, crooked, and sharp Knife. Neither is it convenient to apply the Actual Cautery to stop the Hemorrhage, because it is apt to break forth again anew, when the Escar is fall'n off,

When the Tumour is not as yet ulcerated, a Crucial Incision may be made in the Skin, without penetrating into the Glandulous Bodies; then the four Pieces of the Glandules being separated, the Cancerous Tumour may be held with the Forceps, and afterward cut off. If there be any Vessels swell'd, they may be bound before the Tumour is taken away; but if the Tumour sticks close to the Ribs, the Operation is not usually undertaken.

* * * * *

{227}

CHAP. IX.

Of the Operation of the Empyema.

This Operation is perform'd when it may be reasonably concluded that some corrupt Matter is lodg'd in the Breast, which may be perceiv'd by the weight that the Patient feels in fetching his Breath; being also sensible of the floating of the Matter when he turns himself from one side to another.

If the Tumour appears on the outside, the Abcess may be open'd between the Ribs; but if no external Signs are discern'd, the Surgeon may choose a more convenient place to make the Opening. Thus when the Patient is set upon his Bed, and conveniently supported, the Opening is to be made between the second and third of the Spurious Ribs, within four Fingers breadth of the Spine, and the lower Corner of the Omoplata; to this purpose the Skin is to be taken up a-cross, to cut it in its length, the Surgeon holding it on one side, and the Assistant on the other. The Incision is made with a streight Knife two or three Fingers breadth long, and the Fibres of the great Dorsal-Muscle are cut a-cross, that they may not stop the Opening. Then the Surgeon puts the Fore-Finger of his Left-hand into the Incision, to remove the Fibres, and divides the Intercostal Muscles, guiding the Point of the Knife with his Finger to pierce the Pleuron, for fear of wounding {228} the Lungs, which sometimes adhere thereto, the Opening being thus finish'd, if the Matter runs well, it must be taken out; but if not, the Fore-Finger must be put into the Wound, to disjoyn those Parts of the Lungs that stick to the Pleuron.

To let out the Matter, the Patient must be oblig'd to lean on one side, stopping his Mouth and Nose, and puffing up his Cheeks, as if he were to blow vehemently; then if Blood appears, a greater quantity of it may be taken away than if it were Matter, in regard that a Flux of Matter weakens more than that of Blood. It is also worth the while to observe, that in making the Incision, the Intercostal Muscles ought to be cut a-cross, that the side of the Ribs may not be laid bare, by which means the Wound will not so soon become Fistulous.

If it be judg'd that purulent Matter is contain'd in both sides of the Breast, it is requisite that the Operation be done on each side; it being well known that the Breast is divided into two Parts by the Mediastinum: But in this case the two Holes made by the Incision must not be left open at the same time, for fear of suffocating the Patient.

The Dressing and Bandage.

The Wound is dress'd with a Tent of Lint arm'd with Balsam, being soft, and blunt at the end, which enters only between the Ribs, for fear of hurting the Lungs; but a good Pledget of Lint is more convenient than a Linnen {229} Tent, however a Thread must be ty'd to the Pledget or Tent, lest it shou'd fall into the Breast; and Bolsters are to be put into the Wound; as also a Plaister or Band over the whole. This Dressing is to be kept close with a Napkin fasten'd round the Breast with Pins, and supported by a Scapulary, which is a sort of Band, the breadth of which is equal to that of six Fingers, having a Hole in the middle to let in the Head: One of its ends falls behind and the other before; and they are both fasten'd to the Napkin. Thus the Patient is laid in Bed, and set half upright. If the Lungs hinder the running out of the Matter, a Pipe is us'd, and the Wound afterward dress'd according to Art.

* * * * *

CHAP. X.

Of the Operation of the Paracentesis of the Lower-Belly.

This Manual Operation is sometimes necessary in a Dropsie, when Watry Humours are contain'd in the Cavity of the Belly, or else between the Teguments. The Disease is manifest by the great Swelling; and the Operation is perform'd with a Cane, or a Pipe made of Silver or Steel, with a sharp Stilet at the end; altho' the Ancients were wont to do it with a Lancet. The Patient being supported, sitting on a Bed, or in a great Elbow-Chair, to the end that the Water may run downward, {230} a Servant must press the Belly with his Hands, that the Tumour may be extended, whilst the Surgeon perforates it three or four Fingers breadth below the Navel, and makes the Puncture on the side, to avoid the White-Line; but before the Opening is made, it is expedient that the Skin be a little lifted up. The pointed Stilet being accompany'd with its Pipe, remains in the Part after the Puncture; but it is remov'd to let out the Water; and a convenient quantity of it is taken away, accordingly as the Strength of the Patient will admit. The Stilet makes so small an Opening, that it is not to be fear'd lest the Water shou'd run out, which might happen in making use of the Lancet, because there wou'd be occasion for a thicker Pipe. When a new Puncture is requisite, it must be begun beneath the former; but if the Waters cause the Navel to stand out, the Opening may be made therein, without seeking for any other place.

The Bandage and Dressing

Are prepar'd with a large four-double Bolster kept close with a Napkin folded into three or four Folds, which is in like manner supported by the Scapulary.

The Operation of the Paracentesis of the Scrotum_

Is undertaken when those Parts are full of Water, after this manner: Assoon as the Patient is plac'd in a convenient Posture, either {231} standing or sitting, the Operator lays hold on the Scrotum with one Hand, presseth it a little to render the Tumour hard, and makes a Puncture, as in the Paracentesis of the Abdomen. In an Hydrocele that happens to young Infants, the Opening may be made with a Lancet, to take away all the Water at once: But in Men, especially when there is a great quantity thereof, it is more expedient to do it with the sharp-pointed Pipe; but the Testicles are to be drawn back, for fear of wounding 'em with the Point of the Instrument.

If the Hydrocele be apparently Encysted, the Membrane containing the Water is to be consum'd with Causticks, which is done by laying a Cautery in the place where the Incision shou'd be made, and afterward opening the Escar with a Lancet.

When the Puncture is made, it ought to be done in the upper-part of the Scrotum, because it is less painful than the lower, and less subject to Inflammation.

* * * * *

CHAP XI.

Of the Operation of Gastroraphy.

This Operation is usually perform'd when there is a Wound in the Belly so wide as to let out the Entrails. If there be a considerable Wound in the Intestine, it may be sow'd up with the Glover's Stitch, the manner of making which we have before explain'd. If {232} the Omentum or Caul be mortify'd, the corrupted Part must be cut off; to which purpose it is requisite to take a Needle with waxed Thread, and to pass it into the sound Part a-cross the Caul, without pricking the Vessels. Then the Caul being ty'd on both sides with each of the Threads that have been pass'd double, may be cut an Inch below the Ligature, and the Threads will go thro' the Wound, so as to be taken away after the Suppuration. Afterward the Intestines are to be put up again into the Belly, by thrusting 'em alternately with the end of the Fingers. But if they cannot be restor'd to their proper Place without much difficulty, Spirituous Fomentations may be made with an handful of the Flowers of Camomile and Melilot, an Ounce of Anise, with as much Fennel and Cummin-Seeds; half an

Ounce of Cloves and Nutmegs: Let the whole Mass be boil'd in Milk, adding an Ounce of Camphirated Spirit of Wine, and two Drams of Saccharum Saturni, with two Scruples of Oil of Anise, and bathe the Entrails with this Fomentation very hot. Otherwise,

Apply Animals cut open alive; or else boil Skeins of raw Thread in Milk, and foment 'em with this Decoction in like manner very hot.

Before the Suture of Stitching of the Intestines is made, it is expedient to foment 'em with Spirit of Wine, in which a little Camphire hath been dissolv'd: But if they be mortify'd, they must not be sown up again, but fomented with Spirituous Liquors. No Clysters are to be given to the Patient, for fear {233} causing the Intestine to swell; but a Suppository may be apply'd: Or else he may make use of a Laxative Diet-Drink, if it be necessary to open his Body: He ought also to be very temperate and abstemious during the Cure, so as to take no other Sustenance than Broths and Gellies.

If the Intestines cannot be put up again, the Wound is to be dilated, avoiding the White-Line, and that too at the bottom rather than at the Top, if it be above. To this purpose the Intestines are to be rank'd along the side of the Wound, and a Bolster is to be laid upon 'em dipt in warm Wine, which may be held by some Assistant. Then the Surgeon introduceth a channel'd Probe into the Belly, and takes a great deal of care to fix the Intestine between the Probe and the   Peritoneum, which may be effected by drawing out the Intestine a little; then holding the Probe with his Left-hand, to fit a crooked Incision-Knife in its chanelling, he cuts the Teguments equally both on the outside and within, and thrusts back the Entrails alternately into the Wound with his Fore-Finger.

The Stitch must be intermitted, being made with two crooked Needles threaded at each end with the same Thread. The Surgeon having at first put the Fore-Finger of his Left-Hand into the Belly, to retain the   Peritoneum, Muscles, and Skin on the side of the Wound, passeth the Needle with his other Hand into the Belly, the Point of which is guided with the Fore-Finger, and penetrates very far: Then he likewise passeth the other {234} Needle thro' the other Lip of the Wound into the Belly, observing the same thing as in the former, and without taking his Fingers off from the Belly. If there are many Points or Stitches to be made, they may be done after the same manner, without removing the Fingers from the Part, whilst a Servant draws together the Lips of the Wound, and ties the Knots. Afterward the Wound may be dress'd, and the Preparatives or Dressings kept close to the Part with the Napkin and Scapulary. But the Patient must be oblig'd to lie on his Belly for some Days successively, to cicatrize the Wound thereof, or that of the Entrails.

If the Intestine were entirely cut, it wou'd be requisite to sow it up round about the Wound, after such a manner that some part of it may always remain open; for if the Patient shou'd recover, his Excrements might be voided thro' the Wound; of which Accident we have an Example in a Soldier belonging to the Hospital Des Invalides at Paris, who liv'd a long time in this Condition.

* * * * *

CHAP. XII.

Of the Operation of the Exomphalus.

This Operation is necessary when the Intestines or Entrails have made a kind of Rupture in the Navel, and may be perform'd thus: When the Patient is laid upon his Back, an Incision is to be made on the Tumour to {235} the Fat, by griping the Skin, if it be possible, or else it may be done without taking it up. Then the Membranes are to be divided with a Fleam to lay open the Peritoneum, for fear of cutting the Intestine; and as soon as the Peritoneum appears, it may be drawn upward with the Nails, in order to make a small Opening therein with some cutting Instrument: Whereupon the Surgeon having put the Fore-Finger of his Left-Hand into the Belly to guide the Point of the Sizzers, with which the Incision is enlarg'd, restores the Intestine to its proper Place, and loosens the Caul if it stick to the Tumour: But if the Entrails are fasten'd to the Caul, it is requisite to separate 'em by cutting a little of the Caul, rather than to touch the Intestine; which last being reduc'd, a Servant may press the Belly on the side of the Wound; so that if a Mass of Flesh be found in the Caul, which hath been form'd by the sticking of the Caul to the Muscles and Peritoneum, this Fleshy Mass must be entirely loosen'd, and then a Ligature may be made to take it away, with some part of the Caul, as we have already shewn in the Gastroraphy. Afterward the Stitch is to be made, as in that Operation, and the Wound must be dress'd, observing the same Precautions. The Dressing is to be supported in like manner with the Napkin and Scapulary.

* * * * *

{236}

CHAP. XIII.

Of the Operation of the Bubonocele, and of the compleat Rupture.

When the Intestinal Parts are fall'n into the Groin or the Scrotum, the Operation of the Bubonocele may be conveniently perform'd; to which purpose the Patient is to be laid upon his Back, with his Buttocks somewhat high; then the Skin being grip'd a-cross the Tumour, the Surgeon holds it on one side, and the Assistant on the other, till he makes an Incision, following the Folds or Wrinkles of the Groin; when the Fat appears, it is requisite to tear off either with a Fleam or even with the Nails, every thing that lies in the way, till the Intestine be laid open, which must be drawn out a little, to see if it do not cleave to the Rings of the Muscles. The Intestine must be gently handl'd, to dissolve the Excrements; and those Parts must be afterward put up again into the Belly (if it be possible) with the two Fore-Fingers, thrusting 'em alternately; but if they cannot be reduc'd, the Wound is to be dilated upward, by introducing a channell'd Probe into the Belly, to let the Sizzers into its Channelling. If the Probe cannot enter, the Intestine must be taken out a little, laying a Finger upon it near the Ring, and making a small Scarification in the Ring, with a streight Incision-Knife guided with the {237} Finger, to let in the Probe, into which may be put a crooked Knife, to cut the Ring; that is to say, to dilate the Wound on the inside; but care must be had to avoid penetrating too far, for fear of dividing a Branch of Arteries; and then the Parts may be put up into the Belly. If the Caul had caus'd the Rupture, it wou'd be requisite to bind it, and to cut off whatsoever is corrupted, scarifying the Ring on the inside, to make a good Cicatrice or Scar.

The Dressing and Bandage.

The Dressing may be prepar'd with a Linnen-Tent, soft and blunt, of a sufficient thickness and length, to hinder the Intestines from re-entring into the Rings by their Impulsion, a Thread being ty'd thereto, to draw it out as occasion serves. Then Pledgets are to be put into the Wound, after they have been dipt in a good Digestive, such as Turpentine with the Yolk of an Egg, applying at the same time a Plaister, a Bolster of a Triangular Figure, and the Bandage call'd Spica, which is made much after the same manner as that which is us'd in the Fracture of the Clavicle.

Of the compleat Hernia or Rupture.

It happens when the Intestinal Parts fall into the Scrotum in Men, or into the bottom of the Lips of the Matrix in Women. To perform this Operation, the Patient must be laid upon his Back, as in the Bubonocele, and the Incision carry'd on after the same manner; which is to {238} be made in the Scrotum, tearing off the Membranes to the Intestine. Then a Search will be requisite, to observe whether any parts stick to the Testicle; if the Caul doth so, it must be taken off, leaving a little Piece on the Testicle; but if it be the Intestine, so that those Parts cannot be separated without hurting one of 'em, it is more expedient to impair the Testicle than the Intestine. If the Caul be corrupted, it must be cut to the sound Part, and the Wound is to be dress'd with Pledgets, Bolsters, and the Bandage Spica; as in the Bubonocele.

* * * * *

CHAP. XIV.

Of the Operation of Castration.

The Mortification or the Sarcocele of the Testicles, gives occasion to this Operation; to perform which, the Patient must be laid upon his Back, with his Buttocks higher than his Head, his Legs being kept open, and the Skin of the Scrotum taken up, one end of which is to be held by a Servant, and the other by the Surgeon, who having made a longitudinal Incision therein, or from the top to the bottom, slips off the Flesh of the Dartos which covers the Testicle, binds up the Vessels that lie between the Rings and the Tumour, and cuts 'em off a Fingers breadth beneath the Ligature: But care must be taken to avoid tying the Spermatick Vessels too hard, for fear of a Convulsion, and {239} to let one end of the Thread pass without the Wound. If an Excrescence of Flesh stick to the Testicle, and it be moveable or loose, it is requisite to take it off neatly, leaving a small Piece of it on the Testicle; and if any considerable Vessels appear in the Tumour, they must be bound before they are cut.

The Dressing and Bandage.

The Dressing is made with Pledgets and Bolsters laid upon the Scrotum; and the proper Bandage is the Suspensor of the Scrotum, which hath four Heads or Ends, of which the upper serve as a Cincture or Girdle; and the lower passing between the Thighs, and fasten'd behind to the Cincture.

There is also another Bandage of the Scrotum, having in like manner four Heads, of which the upper constitute the Cincture; but it is slit at the bottom, and hath no Seams; the lower Heads crossing one another, to pass between the Thighs, and to be join'd to the Cincture. Both these sorts of Bandages have a Hole to give Passage to the Yard.

* * * * *

{240}

CHAP. XV.

Of the Operation of the Stone in the Ureter.

If the Stone be stopt at the Sphincter of the Bladder, it ought to be thrust back with a Probe: If it stick at the end of the Glans, it may be press'd to let it out; and if it cannot come forth, a small Incision may be made in the opening of the Glans on its side.

But if the Stone be remote from the Glans, it is requisite to make an Incision into the Ureter; to which purpose, the Surgeon having caus'd the Skin to be drawn upward, holds the Yard between two Fingers, making a Longitudinal Incision on its side upon the Stone, which must be prest between the Fingers to cause it to fly out; or else it may be taken out with an Extractor. Then if the Incision were very small, the Skin needs only to be let go, and it will heal of it self; but if it were large, a small Leaden Pipe is to be put into the Ureter, lest it shou'd be altogether clos'd up by the Scar: It is also expedient to anoint the

Pipe with some Desiccative Medicine, and to dress the Wound with Balsam. Afterward a little Linnen-Bag or Case is to be made, in which the Yard is to be put, to keep on the Dressing; but it must be pierc'd at the end, for the convenience of making Water, having two Bands at the other end, which are ty'd round about the Waste.

* * * * *

{241}

CHAP. XVI.

Of the Operation of Lithotomy.

This Operation is undertaken when it is certainly known that there is a Stone in the Bladder; to be assur'd of which, it may not be improper to introduce a Finger into the Anus near the Os Pubis, by which means the Stone is sometimes felt, if there be any: The Finger is likewise usually put into the Anus of young Virgins, and into the Vagina Uteri of Women, for the same purpose. But it is more expedient to make use of the Probe, anointed with Grease, after this manner: The Patient being laid on his Back, the Operator holds the Yard streight upward, the Glans lying open between his Thumb and Fore-finger; then holding the Probe with his Right-hand on the side of the Rings, he guides it into the Yard, and when it is enter'd, turns the Handle toward the Pubes, drawing out the Yard a little, to the end that the Canal of the Ureter may lie streight. If it be perceiv'd that the Probe hath not as yet pass'd into the Bladder, a Finger is to be put into the Anus, to conduct it thither. Afterward in order to know whether a Stone be lodg'd in the Bladder, the Probe ought to be shaken a little therein, first on the Right-side, and then on the Left; and if a small Noise be heard, it may be concluded for certain that there is a Stone: But if it be judg'd that the {242} Stone swims in the Bladder, so that it cannot be felt, the Patient must be oblig'd to make Water with a hollow Probe.

Another manner of searching may be practis'd thus: Let the Yard be rais'd upward, inclining a little to the side of the Belly; let the Rings of the Probe be turn'd upon the Belly, and the end on the side of the Anus; and then let this Instrument be introduc'd, shaking it a little on both sides, to discover the

Stone.

In order to perform the Operation of Lithotomy, the Patient must be laid along upon a Table of a convenient height, so as that the Surgeon may go about his Work standing; the Patient's Back must also lean upon the Back of a Chair laid down, and trimm'd with Linnen-Cloth, lest it shou'd hurt his Body; his Legs must be kept asunder, and the Soles of his Feet on the sides of the Table, whilst a Man gets up behind him to hold his Shoulders: His Arms and Legs must be also bound with Straps or Bands. Then a channell'd Probe being put up into the Bladder, a Servant standing upon the Table on the side of the Chair, holds the Back of the Instrument between his two Fore-fingers on that Part of the Perinem where the Incision ought to be begun, which is to be made between his Fingers with a sharp Knife that cuts on both sides: The Incision may be three or four Fingers breadth on the left side of the Raphe or Suture: But in Children its length must not exceed two Fingers breadth. If the Incision were too little to give Passage to the Stone, it wou'd be more expedient to enlarge it than to stretch the Wound {243} with the Dilatators. When the Convex Part where the channelling of the Probe lies, shall be well laid open, the Conductors may be slipt into the same Channelling, between which the Forceps is to be put, having before taken away the Probe. Some Operators make use of a Gorgeret or Introductor to that purpose, conveying the end of it into the Chanelling of the Probe; which is remov'd to introduce the Forceps into the Bladder: And as soon as they are fixt therein, the Conductors or Gorgeret must be likewise taken out. Afterward search being made for the Stone, it must be held fast, and drawn out of the Bladder: But if the Stone be long, and the Operator hath got hold thereof by the two Ends, he must endeavour to lay hold on it again by the Middle, to avoid the great scattering which wou'd happen in the Passage. The Stones are also sometimes so large, that there is an absolute necessity of leaving 'em in the Bladder. Again, if the Stone sticks very close to the Bladder, the Extraction ought to be deferr'd for some time; and perhaps it may be loosen'd in the Suppuration. Lastly, when the Stone hath been taken out, an Extractor is usually introduc'd into the Bladder, to remove the Gravel, Fragments, and Clots of Blood.

After the Operation, the Patient is carry'd to his Bed, having before cover'd the Wound with a good Bolster; and if an Hemorrhage happens, it is to be stopt with Astringents. A Tent must also be put into the Wound, when it is suspected that some Stone or Gravel may as yet remain therein: But if it evidently appears that {244} there is none, the Wound may be dress'd with Pledgets, a Plaister, and a Bolster, of a Figure convenient for the Part. The Dressing may be staid with a Sling supported by a Scapulary; or else the Bandage of the double T. may be us'd, the manner of the Application of which we have shewn elsewhere. The Patient's Thighs must be drawn close to one another, and ty'd with a small Band, lest they shou'd be set asunder again.

The Operation of Lithotomy in Women is usually perform'd by the lesser Preparative, which is done by putting the Fore-finger and Middle-finger into the Vagina Uteri, or into the Rectum in young Virgins, to draw the Stone to the Neck of the Bladder, and keep it steady, so that it may be taken out with a Hook, or other Instrument.

This Operation may also be effected in Women, almost in the same manner as in Men; for after having caus'd the Female Patient to be set in the same Posture or Situation as the Men are usually plac'd, according to the preceeding Description, the Conductors may be convey'd into the Ureter, to let in the Forceps between 'em, with which the Stone may be drawn out: But if it be too thick, a small Incision is to be made in the Right and Left side of the Ureter.

The lesser Preparative was formerly us'd in the Lithotomy of Men, after this manner: The Finger was put into the Anus, to draw the Stone toward the Perinem; then an Incision was made upon the Stone on the side of the Suture, and it was taken out with an Instrument.

* * * * *

{245}

CHAP. XVII.

Of the Operation of the Puncture of the Perinem.

This Operation is necessary in a Suppression of Urine, where the Inflammation is so great, that the Probe cannot be introduc'd. Then an

Incision is to be made with the Knife or Lancet, in the same Place where it is done in Lithotomy; and a small Tube or Pipe is to be put in the Bladder, till the Inflammation be remov'd.

* * * * *

CHAP. XVIII.

Of the Operation of the Fistula in Ano.

Fistula's are callous Ulcers: If one of these happen in the Fundament, and is open on the outside, it may be cur'd thus: After the Patient hath been laid upon his Belly on the side of a Bed, with his Legs asunder, the Surgeon makes a small Incision with his Knife in the Orifice of the Fistula, in order to pass therein another small crooked Incision-Knife, at the end of which is a Pointed Stilet with a little Silver Head which covers it, to the end that it may enter without causing Pain. When the Surgeon hath convey'd his Knife into the {246} Fistula, having the Fore-finger of his Left-hand in the Anus or Fundament, he pulls off its Head, holding the Handle with one Hand, and the Stilet that pierceth the Anus with the other; and at last draws out the Instrument to cut the Fistula entirely at one Stroke.

If the Fistula hath an Opening into the Intestine, an Incision is to be made on the outside at the Bottom thereof, to open it in the Place where a small Tumour or Inflammation usually appears, or else in the Place where the Patient feels a Pain when it is touch'd. If the Tumour be remote from the Anus, it may be open'd with the Potential Cautery, to avoid a greater Inconvenience. After having thus laid open the very bottom, the little Incision-Knife and Stilet, with its Head, is to be pass'd therein, the end of the Stilet is to be drawn thro' the Anus, and the Flesh is to be cut all at once. But if the Fistula be situated too far forward in the Fundament, the Sphincter of the Anus must not be entirely cut, otherwise the Excrements cannot be any longer retain'd. Lastly, when the Fistula hath been treated after this manner, all its Sinuosities or Winding-Passages ought likewise to be open'd, and the Wound being fill'd with thick Pledgets steept in some Anodyn, is to be cover'd with a Plaister and a Triangular Bolster; as also with the Bandage call'd the T.

* * * * *

CHAP. XIX.

Of the Suture or Stitching of a Tendon.

It is requisite to undertake this Operation when the Tendons are cut, and when they become very thick. If the Wound be heal'd, it must be open'd again to discover the Tendon, and the Part must be bended, to draw together again the ends of the Tendons. Then the Surgeon taking a flat, streight, and fine Needle, with a double waxed Thread, passeth it into a small Bolster, and makes a Knot at the end of the Thread, to be stopt upon the Bolster. Afterward he pierceth the Tendon from the outside to the inside, at a good distance, lest the Thread shou'd tear it, and proceeds to pass the Needle in like manner under the other end of the Tendon, upon which is laid a small Bolster, for the Thread to be ty'd in a Knot over it. Then he causeth the Extremities of the Tendons to lie a little one upon another, by bending the Part, and dresseth the Wound with some Balsam. It may not be improper here to observe, that Ointments are never to be apply'd to the Tendons, which wou'd cause 'em to putrifie, but altogether Spirituous Medicaments; and that the Part must be bound up, lest the Extension of it shou'd separate the Tendons.

* * * * *

CHAP. XX.

Of the Caesarian Operation.

When a Woman cannot be deliver'd by the ordinary means, this bold and dangerous Operation hath been sometimes perform'd with good Success. The Woman being laid upon her Back, the Surgeon makes a Longitudinal Incision beneath the Navel, on the side of the White-Line, till the Matrixappears, which he openeth, taking great care to avoid wounding the Child: Then he divides the Membranes with which it is wrapt up, separates the After-Burden from the Matrix, and takes out the Child. Lastly he washeth the Wound with warm Wine, and dispatcheth the Gastroraphy or Stitching up of the Belly, without sowing the Matrix. After the Operation, Injections are to be made into the Matrix, to cause a Flux of Blood; and a pierc'd Pessary must be introduc'd into its Neck.

* * * * *

{249}

CHAP. XXI.

Of the Operation of Amputation, with its proper Dressings and Bandages.

The Leg is usually cut off at the Ham; the Thigh as near as can be to the Knee; and the Arm as near as is possible to the Wrist: But an Amputation is never made in a Joynt, except in the Fingers and Toes.

In order to cut off a Leg, the Patient is to be set on the side of his Bed, or in a Chair, and supported by divers Assistants; one of 'em being employ'd to hold the Leg at the bottom, and another to draw the Skin upward above the Knee, to the end that the Flesh may cover the Bone again after the Operation. In the mean while a very thick Bolster is laid under the Ham, upon which are made two Ligatures, viz. the first above the Knee, to stop the Blood, by screwing it up with the Tourniquet or Gripe-Stick; and the second below the Knee, to render the Flesh firm for the Knife. Before the Ligature is drawn close with the Gripe-Stick, a little piece of Paste-board is to be put underneath, for fear of pinching the Skin. Thus the Leg being well fixt, the Surgeon placeth himself between both the Legs of the Patient, to make the Incision with a crooked Knife, turning it circularly to the Bone, and laying one Hand upon the Back of the Knife, which must have no Edge. Afterward the Periosteum is to be {250} scrap'd with an Incision-Knife, and the Flesh with the Vessels that lie between the two Bones are to be cut. When the Flesh is thus separated, a Cleft Band is to be laid upon it, with which the Heads are cross'd, to draw the Flesh upward, to the intent that the Bones may be cut farther, and that it may cover 'em after the Amputation, as also to facilitate the Passage of the Saw. Then the Surgeon holds the Leg with his Left-hand, and saweth with his Right, which he lets fall upon the two Bones, to divide 'em asunder at the same time, beginning with the Perone or Fibula, and ending with the Tibia. But it is necessary to incline the Saw, and to go gently in the beginning, to make way for it, and afterward to work it faster. The Leg being cut off, the Ligature must be unty'd below the Knee, loosening the Gripe-Stick, to let the Blood run a little, and to discern the Vessels with greater facility; and then the Gripe-Stick may be twisted again, to stop the Blood; which some Surgeons effect, by laying Pieces of Vitriol upon the Opening of the Arteries, and Astringent Powders, on a large Bolster of Cotton or Tow, to be apply'd to the end of the Stump; but if such a method be us'd, it is requisite that some Person be employ'd to keep on the whole Dressing with his Hand during twenty four Hours. However this Custom hath prevail'd in the Hospital of Hotel-Dieu at Paris.

Others make a Ligature of the Vessels, taking up the ends of 'em with a pair of Forceps, having a Spring; or with the Valet a Patin, which is a sort of Pincers that are clos'd with a small {251} Ring let down to the bottom of the Branches. These Pincers being held by a Servant, the Surgeon passeth a Needle with wax'd Thread, into the Flesh, below the Vessel, bringing it back again, and with the two ends of the Thread makes a good Ligature upon the same Vessel; then he looseth the Gripe-Stick and the Band, the Stump is to be somewhat bended, and the Flesh let down to cover the Bones.

The Dressing and Bandage.

After the Operation, it is requisite to lay small Bolsters upon the Vessels, and dry Pledgets upon the two Bones, as also many other Folds of Linnen strew'd with Astringent Powders; and over all another large Bolster or Pledget of Cotton or Tow, cover'd in like manner with Astringent Powders; then the whole Dressing is to be wrapt up with a Plaister and a Bolster, in form of a Malta Cross; so that there are three or four Longitudinal Bolsters, and one Circular.

The Surgeon usually begins to apply the Malta Cross and Bolster under the Ham, crossing the Heads or Ends upon the Stump, and causeth 'em to be held by a Servant that Supports the Part; then he likewise crosseth the other Heads, and layeth on the two Longitudinal Bolsters that cross each other in the middle of the Stump, together with a third Longitudinal, which is brought round about the Stump, to stay the two former: These Bolsters ought to be three Fingers broad, and very long, to pass over the Stump. Afterward he proceeds to apply, {252}

The Bandage commonly call'd Capeline by French Surgeons, or the Head-Bandage.

Which is prepar'd with a Band four Ells long, and three Fingers broad, roll'd up with one Ball, three Circumvolutions being made on the side of the cut Part, the Band is to be carry'd upward with Rollers, passing obliquely above the Knee; and is brought down again along its former Turns; If it be thought fit to make this Bandage with the same Band, it must be let down to the middle of the cut Part, and carry'd up again to the Knee, many back-folds being made, which are stay'd with the Circumvolutions, till the Stump be entirely covered, and the whole Bandage wrapt up with Rollers or Bolsters.

The Capeline or Head-Bandage, having two Heads, is made with a Band of the same breadth, but somewhat longer. This Band being at first apply'd to the middle of the cut Part or Wound, the Heads are carry'd up above the Knee; and one of the Ends are turn'd backward, to bring it down, and to pass it over the end of the Stump. At every back-fold which is form'd above and below the Knee, a Circumvolution is to be made with the other end of the Band, to strengthen the back-folds, continuing to bring the Band downward and upward, till the whole Stump be cover'd: Then Rollers are made round about the Stump, and the Band is stay'd above the Knee. Afterward the Part may be brought to Suppuration, cleans'd and cicatriz'd.

* * * * *

{253}

CHAP. XXII.

Of the Operation of the Aneurism.

This Operation is perform'd when the Surgeon hath prickt an Artery, or when a Tumour ariseth in an Artery.

To this purpose the Patient is set in a Chair, and a Servant employ'd in holding his Arm in a Posture proper for the Operation; then a Bolster is to be laid four double, following the Progress of the Artery, to the end that the Ligature may better press the Vessel; and the Arm may be also surrounded with another single Bolster, on which is made a Ligature screw'd up with a Gripe-Stick, provided the Arm be not too much swell'd; for in this Case it wou'd be more expedient to deferr the Operation for fear of a Gangrene. The Artery being thus well stopt, the Surgeon lays hold on the Arm with one Hand, below the Tumour, and with the other makes an Incision with his Lancet, beginning at the bottom of the Tumour, and ending on the top along the Progress of the Artery. When the Tumour is open'd, the coagulated Blood may be discharg'd with a Finger; and if there are any Strings at the bottom, they may be cut with a crooked Pair of Sizzers, to the end that all the Clods of Blood, and other extraneous Bodies which are sometimes form'd in Aneurisms when they are very inveterate may be more {254} easily remov'd. But the Gripe-Stick must be loosen'd, to discover the Opening of the Artery with greater facility, and the Artery separated from the Membranes with a Fleam; for it wou'd be dangerous to cut it with a streight Incision-Knife: The Artery must also be supported with a convenient Instrument to divide it from the Nerve and Membranes; and to be assur'd of the Place of its Opening, the Gripe-Stick may be somewhat loosen'd, and afterward screw'd up again. In the mean time the Surgeon gives the Instrument to a Servant to hold, whilst he passeth under the Artery a crooked Needle with a wax'd String, cuts the Thread, and takes away the Needle: Then he begins to make the Ligature beneath the Opening of the Artery, tying at first a single Knot, on which may be put (if you please) a small Bolster, that may be kept steady with two other Knots: It is also necessary that another Ligature be made in the lower part of the Artery, by reason that the little lateral Arteries might otherwise let out Blood.

The Artery ought not to be cut between the two Ligatures, lest the first Ligature shou'd be forc'd by the Impulsion of the Blood; but the Thread must be let fall, that it may rot with the Suppuration. Then the Wound may be dress'd with Pledgets, Bolsters strew'd with Astringent Powders and a Plaister; a Bolster being also laid in the Fold of the Elbow. {255}

The Bandage

Is made with a Band six Ells long, and an Inch broad, roll'd with one end, being at first apply'd with divers Circumvolutions under the Elbow, and moderately bound. Many turns are to be made, and a thick and streight Bolster, is to be laid upon the Tumour, (as in the Bandage for Phlebotomy) along the Artery, till it pass under the Arm-Hole: The Arm and Bolster must be surrounded with the Band, which is brought up with small Rollers, to the Arm-Pit, and stay'd with Circumvolutions round about the Breast. Afterward the Patient is to be laid in his Bed, with the Arm lying somewhat bended on the Pillow, and the Hand a little higher than the Elbow.

* * * * *

CHAP. XXIII.

Of the Operation of Phlebotomy.

To perform this Operation, the Surgeon holds the Lancet between his Thumb and Fore-finger, and three other Fingers lying upon the Patient's Arm, and thrusts the Point of the lancet into the Vessel, carrying the same Point somewhat upward, to make the Orifice the greater. If a Tendon, which is known by its hardness; or an Artery, which is discover'd by Pulsation, appear beyond the Vein, and very near it, the Lancet must be only set very {256} forward in the Vein, and drawn back again streight, without turning it up, otherwise the Artery or Tendon wou'd be certainly cut with the Point. If the Artery or Tendon lies immediately under the Vein, the later must be prickt somewhat underneath, holding the Lancet inclin'd side-ways, and thrusting it very little forward; so that the Point will finish the Opening, by turning it upward.

If the Artery stick too close to the Vein, the later is to be prickt higher or lower than it is ordinarily done; and if the Vein be superficial, and lie close upon a hard Muscle, the Lancet must not be thrust downright into the Vein, but it is requisite to carry it somewhat obliquely, and to take the Vessel above, lest the Muscle and its Membrane shou'd be prickt, which wou'd cause a great deal of Pain, and perhaps a vehement Inflammation. It is well known that the Veins of the Right Arm are usually open'd with the Right-hand, and those of the Left-Arm with the Left-hand.

The Bandage

Is made thus: The Surgeon having laid a Bolster upon the Orifice, keeps it close with two Fingers, and holds the Band or Fillet with the other Hand; then taking one end of the Fillet with the Middle-Finger, Fore-Finger, and Thumb, and applying it to the Bolster, he makes with the longest end of the Fillet divers Figures in form of the Letters KY in the Fold of the Arm; as also a back-fold with the shorter end of the Fillet, held between three {257} Fingers. Afterward both ends of the Fillet are ty'd beneath the Elbow.

If an Inflammation happens after the Operation, the Bolsters are to be dipt in Oxycratum: but if the Orifice were so small as to produce a Rhombus, it wou'd be requisite to press the Wound often with two Fingers, and immediately to apply a Bolster dipt in Oxycratum.

* * * * *

CHAP. XXIV.

Of the Operation of Encysted Tumours.

If the Tumours are small and hanging, and have a narrow bottom, a Ligature may be made with Horse-Hair or Silk, dipt in Aqua-Fortis, which will cause 'em to fall off of themselves after some time; or else they may be cut above the Ligature.

If the Tumour or Wen be thick, and its bottom large, a Crucial Incision is to be made in the Skin, without impairing the Cystis or Bagg; and when the Incision is finish'd, the Bag may be torn off with the Nails, or with the Handle of a Pen-Knife; but sometimes it is necessary to dissect it. If there be any considerable Vessels at the Root, they may be bound, or else cut; and the Blood may be stopt with Astringents. If any parts of the Cystis remain, they are to be consum'd with Corrosives; and the Lips of the Wound are to be drawn together without a Stitch, making use {258} only of an agglutinative Plaister. But if the Tumour adheres very close to the Pericranium, it is most expedient not to meddle with it at all.

Of Ganglions.

Ganglions are Tumours arising upon the Tendons and Nervous Parts, which may be cur'd by thrusting 'em violently, and making a very streight Bandage, provided they be very recent; a resolvent Plaister is to be also apply'd to the Part.

* * * * *

CHAP. XXV.

Of the Operation of the Hydrocephalus.

This Operation is perform'd when it is necessary to discharge watry Humours out of the Head: If these Waters lie under the Skin, a very large Opening is to be made with a Lancet, and a small Tube or Pipe left therein to let 'em run out. If the Water be situated between the Brain and the Dura Mater, the Membrane is to be perforated with a Lancet, after the Trepan hath been apply'd, according to the usual Method, of which we have already given some account: Cauteries and Scarifications may be also us'd to very good purpose in this Disease.

* * * * *

{259}

CHAP. XXVI.

Of the operation of cutting the Tongue-String.

When the Ligament of the Tongue in Infants is extended to its Extremity, they cannot suck without difficulty; and when grown up, they have an impediment in their Speech.

This Ligament may be cut with a little pair of Sizzers; to which purpose the Thumb of the Left-hand being laid upon the Gum of the lower Jaw, to keep the Mouth open, the Tongue may be rais'd upward with the Fore-Finger of the same Hand, and the Sizzers may be pass'd between the two Fingers, to divide the String as near as is possible to the Root of the Tongue, avoiding the Vessels: If an Hemorrhage happens, recourse may be had to Styptick-Waters.

Afterward the Nurse must take care to let a Finger be often put into the Child's Mouth, to prevent the re-uniting of the String.

* * * * *

{260}

CHAP. XXVII.

Of the Operation of opening stopt Ductus's.

If there be only one Membrane that stops the Entrance of the Vagina, an Incision may be made, and a Leaden Pipe put into it, having Rings to fasten it to the Waste, to hinder the re-uniting of the Wound.

If the Lips of the Pudendum are conglutinated or clos'd up, the Patient must be laid upon her Back, and her Knees rais'd up, in order to make an Incision with a crooked Incision-Knife, beginning at the Top; and then a Leaden Pipe is to be put into the Opening.

If the Vagina be fill'd with a Fleshy Substance, an Incision is to be made therein, till it be entirely perforated, putting at the same time a Leaden Tube into the Orifice.

If the Urinary Ductus as well in young Boys as in Virgins, be stopt up, an Incision is to be made therein with a very narrow Lancet; and if a small Leaden Pipe can be conveniently introduc'd, it may be done; but it is not very necessary, in regard that Children are almost always making Water, which wou'd of it self hinder the closing of the Orifice.

If the Ductus of the Ear be stopt with a Membrane, it must be perforated, taking care not to go too far, for fear of piercing the Membrane of the Tympanum or Drum, and {261} a small Leaden Pipe is to be put into the Opening.

If there be a carnous Excrescence on the outside of the Ear, a Ligature ought to be made therein, or else it may be cut with a pair of Sizzers, to cause it to fall off; and the rest of the Fleshy Substance that remains in the Ear must be consum'd with Causticks, convey'd to the Part by the means of a small Tube, care being had, nevertheless, to avoid cauterizing the Tympanum.

* * * * *

CHAP. XXVIII.

Of the Operation of the Phimosis and Paraphimosis.

When the Prutrium is so streight that the Glans can be no longer uncover'd, this Indisposition is call'd Phimosis; but if the Prutriumbe turn'd back above the Glans, after such a manner that it can no longer cover the same Glans, it is a Paraphimosis. If in the Phimosis the Prutrium cleaves very close round about the Glans, it is most expedient to let it alone; but if in handling the Glans it be perceiv'd that it is moveable, or else that some parts of it only stick together, the Operation may be perform'd after this manner: The Patient being set in a Chair, a Servant is employ'd in pulling back the Skin to the Root of the Penis, to the end that the Incision may be {262} made directly at the bottom of the Glans: Then the Surgeon having drawn out the bottom of the Prutium, introduceth a small Instrument with a very sharp Point on its flat side, at the end of which is fixt a Button of Wax, pierceth the Prutium at the bottom of the Glans on the side of the Thread, and finisheth the Incision by drawing the Instrument toward himself.

The Paraphimosis is cur'd by making Fomentations on the Part, to allay the Inflammation if there be any; and it is to be pull'd down with the Fingers. But if Medicinal Preparations prove ineffectual, Scarifications are to be made round about the Prutrium; and afterward convenient Remedies may be apply'd to remove the Inflammation, and prevent the Mortification of the Part; so that at length the Prutium may be drawn over the Glans.

* * * * *

CHAP. XXIX.

Of the Operation of the Varix.

In order to cure this Tumour, the Surgeon having first cut the Skin to discover the dilated Vein, separates it from the Membranes, and passeth underneath a crooked Needle with a double wax'd Thread; then he makes a Ligature both above and below the dilatation of the Vein, opens the dilated Part with a Lancet, to let out the Blood, and applies a convenient Bandage: But without performing this {263} Operation, the Vein might be open'd with a Lancet, to draw out a sufficient quantity of Blood; and then the Varixis to be press'd with a somewhat close Bandage.

* * * * *

CHAP. XXX.

Of the Operation of the Panaritium.

The Panaritium is an Abcess which ariseth at the end of the Fingers; some of these Tumours are only superficial, and others penetrate even under the Periosteum; nevertheless after whatsoever manner the Panaritium may happen, it ought to be open'd on the side of the Finger, that the Tendons may not be hurt. If the Abcess be extended under the Periosteum, the opening must be made on the side, and the Lancet thrust forward to the Bone: Afterward the Pus or corrupt Matter is to be discharg'd, which wou'd cause the Tendons to putrifie, if it shou'd remain too long upon 'em.

The Dressing and Bandage

Are made with a Plaister cut in form of a Malta Cross, which is apply'd at the middle to the end of the Finger, the Heads being cross'd round about. The Bolsters must be also cut in the shape of the Malta Cross, or of a plain Cross only; the Band being a Finger's breadth {264} wide, and long enough to be roll'd about the whole Dressing: It must be pierc'd at one of its ends, and cut the length of three Fingers at the other; so that the two Heads may pass thro' the Hole, to surround the Finger with small Rollers.

* * * * *

CHAP. XXXI.

Of the Reduction of the falling of the Anus.

To reduce the Anus to its proper place when it is fallen, the Patient being laid upon his Belly, with his Buttocks higher than his Head, the Operator gently thrusts back the Roll that forms the Anus with his Fingers dipt in the Oil of Roses: Then he applies the Bolsters steept in some Astringent Liquor, and causeth 'em to be supported with a sort of Bandage, the Nature of which we shall shew in treating of the Fracture of the Coccyx, that is to say, the T. the double T. or else the Sling with four Heads.

* * * * *

{265}

CHAP. XXXII.

Of the Reduction of the falling of the Matrix.

In this Operation, the Patient being laid upon her Back, with her Buttocks rais'd up, Fomentations are to be apply'd to the Part; a Linnen Cloth is to be laid upon the Neck of the fallen Matrix; and it is to be thrust very gently with the Fingers, without using much force. If the Matrix shou'd fall out again, it wou'd be requisite to convey a Pessary into it, after it hath been reduc'd; and to enjoyn the Patient to lie on her Back with her legs a-cross.

* * * * *

CHAP. XXXIII.

Of the Application of the Cautery.

The Cautery is an Ulcer which is made in the Skin, by applying Causticks to it, after this manner:

The Surgeon having moisten'd the Skin for a while with Spittle, or else having caus'd a light Friction to be made with a warm Cloth, applies a perforated Plaister to the Part, and breaks the Cautery-Stone, to be laid in {266} the little Hole, leaving it for a longer or shorter time, accordingly as he knows its Efficacy, or as the Skin is more or less Fine. Afterward he scarifieth the Burn with his Lancet, and puts a Suppurative, or piece of fresh Butter into the Part, till the Escar be fallen off.

The Dressing and Bandage.

After the Application of the Lapis Infernalis, or any other Cautery-Stone, it is necessary to lay over it a Plaister, a Bolster, and a Circular Bandage, which ought to be kept sufficiently close, to press the Stone, after a Pea or little Piece of Orrice-Root, hath been put into the Ulcer to keep it open. Then the Patient is to make use of this Bandage, with which he may dress it himself. Take a piece of very strong Cloth, large enough to roll up the Part without crossing above it: And let three or four Holes be made in one of its sides, as many small Ribbans or Pieces of Tape being sow'd to the other, which may be let into the Holes, as occasion serves, to close the Band.

* * * * *

{267}

CHAP. XXXIV.

Of the Application of Leeches.

It is requisite that the Leeches be taken in clear running Waters, and that they be long and slender, having a little Head, the Back green, with yellow Streaks, and the Belly somewhat reddish. Before they are apply'd, it is also expedient to let 'em purge during some Days in fair Water, fast half a Day in a Box without Water. Afterward the Part being rubb'd or chaf'd with warm Water, Milk, or the Blood of some Fowl, the Opening of the Box is to be set to the Part, or the Leeches themselves laid upon a Cloth; for they will not fasten when taken up with the Fingers. The end of their Tail may be cut with a Pair of Sizzers, to see the Blood run, and to determine its quantity, as also to facilitate their sucking. When you wou'd take 'em away, put Ashes, Salt, or any other sharp thing upon their Head, and they will suddenly desist from their Work; but they are not to be pull'd off by force, lest they shou'd leave their Head or Sting in the Wound, which wou'd be of very dangerous consequence. When they are remov'd, let a little Blood run out, and wash the Part with salt Water. {268}

The Dressing

Is made with a Bolster soakt in some Styptick Water, if the Blood will not otherwise stop; or in Brandy or Aqua-Vit?if there be an Inflammation; and it is to be supported with a Bandage proper for the Part.

* * * * *

CHAP. XXXV.

Of the Application of the Seton.

To perform this Operation, a Cotton or Silk Thread is to be taken, after it hath been dipt in Oil of Roses, and let into a kind of Pack-Needle; then the Patient sitting in a Chair, is to hold up his Head backward, whilst the Surgeon gripes the Skin transversely in the Nape of the Neck with his Fingers, or else takes it up with a Pair of Forceps, and passeth the Needle thro' the Holes of the Forceps, leaving the String in the Skin. As often as the Bolster that covers the Seton is taken off, that part of the String which lies in the Wound is to be drawn out, and cut off.

* * * * *

{269}

CHAP. XXXVI.

Of Scarifications.

Scarifications are to be made more or less deep, accordingly as necessity requires, beginning at the bottom, and carrying them on upward, to avoid being hinder'd by the Hemorrhage. They must also be let one into another, that Strings may not be left in the Skin.

* * * * *

CHAP. XXXVII.

Of the Application of Vesicatories.

Vesicatories are compounded with the Powder of Cantharides or Spanish flies, mixt with very sower Leaven, or else with Turpentine. Before they are apply'd, a light friction is to be made on the Part with a warm cloth, and a greater or lesser quantity is to be laid on, accordingly as the Skin is more or less fine, leaving 'em on the Part about seven or eight Hours; then they are to be taken away, and the Blisters are to be open'd, applying thereto some sort of Spirituous Liquor.

* * * * *

{270}

CHAP. XXXVIII.

Of the Application of Cupping-Glasses.

A Good Friction being first made with warm Clothes, lighted Toe is to be put into the Cupping-Glass, or else a Wax-Candle fasten'd to a Counter, and then it is to be apply'd to the Part till the Fire be extinguish'd, and the Skin swell'd, re-iterating the Operation as often as it is necessary; and afterward laying on a Bolster steept in Spirit of Wine. These are call'd dry Cupping-Glasses: But if you wou'd draw Blood, every thing is to be observ'd that we have now mention'd, besides that Scarifications are to be made, according to the usual manner; and the Cupping-Glass is to be set upon the Scarifications: But when the Cupping-Glass is half full of Blood, it must be taken off to be emptied, and the Application thereof is to be re-iterated, as often as it is required to take away any Blood. Lastly, the Incisions are to be wash'd with some Spirituous Liquor; and a Bandage is to be made convenient for the Part.

* * * * *

{271}

CHAP. XXXIX.

Of the opening of Abcesses or Impostumes.

An Abcess or Impostume ought to be open'd in its most mature part, and in the Bias of the Humours, endeavouring to preserve the Fibres of the Muscles from being cut, unless there be an absolute necessity, avoiding also the great Vessels, Tendons, and Nerves. The Opening must be rather large than small, and not too much press'd in letting out the purulent Matter. If the Skin be thick, as it happens in the Heel, it may be par'd with a Razor; and if the Matter be lodg'd under the Nails, it wou'd be required to scrape 'em with Glass before they are pierc'd.

* * * * *

{272}

A

TREATISE

OF THE

OPERATIONS

OF

FRACTURES.

* * * * *

CHAP. I.

Of the Fracture of the Nose.

When the Fracture is considerable, the Nostrils are stopt up, and the Sense of Smelling is lost. In order to reduce it, the Surgeon takes a little Stick wrapt up in Cotton, and introduceth it into the Nostrils as gently as is possible, to raise up the Bones again, laying the Thumb of his Left-hand upon the Nose, to retain 'em in their place. The Bones being thus set, he proceeds to prepare

The Dressing and Bandage

By conveying into the Nostrils certain Leaden Pipes of a convenient Bigness and Figure, which serve to support the Bones, and to facilitate Respiration. But care is to be had to avoid thrusting 'em up too far, for fear of hurting the sides of the Nose; and they are to be anointed with Oil of Turpentine mixt with Spirit of Wine: These Pipes are also to have little Handles, with which they may be fasten'd to the Cap. If there be no Wound in the Nose, there will be no need of a Bandage; but if the Fracture be accompany'd with a Wound, after having apply'd the proper Medicines, it wou'd be requisite to lay upon each side of the Nose a Triangular Bolster, cover'd with a little piece of Paste-board of the same Figure. This small Dressing is to be supported with a kind of Sling that hath four Heads; being a piece of Linnen-Cloath, two Fingers broad, and half an Ell long; it is slit at both ends, and all along, only leaving in the middle a Plain of three Fingers, that is to say, a part which is not cut. The Plain of this Sling is to be laid upon the Fracture, causing the upper Heads to pass behind the Nape of the Neck, which are to be brought back again forward; the lower Heads are likewise to be carry'd behind, crossing above the upper, and afterward to be return'd forward. If the Bones of the Nose be not timely reduc'd, a great Deformity soon happens therein, and a Stink caus'd by the Excrescences and Polypus's.

* * * * *

CHAP. II.

Of the Fracture of the lower Jaw.

The Operator at first puts his Fingers into the Patient's Mouth, to press the Prominences of the Bones; and afterward doth the same thing on the outside. If the Bones pass one over another, a small Extension is to be made. If the Teeth be forc'd out of their Place, they are to be reduc'd, and fasten'd to the sound Teeth with a wax'd Thread.

The Dressing and Bandage.

If the Fracture be only on one side, a Bolster sow'd to a piece of Paste-board is to be laid upon the flat side of the Jaw, both being of the Figure and Size of the Jaw it self. The Bandage of this Fracture is call'd Chevestre, i.e. a Cord or Bridle, by the French Surgeons, and is made by taking a Band roll'd with one Head or End, three Ells long, and two Fingers broad; the Application of it is begun with making a Circumvolution round about the Head in passing over the Fore-head; then the Band is let down under the Chin, and carry'd up again upon the Cheek, near the lesser Corner of the Eye in passing over the Fracture; afterward it is rais'd up to the Head, and brought down again under the Chin, {275} to form a Roller or Bolster upon the Fracture: Thus three or four Circumvolutions and Rollers being made upon the Fracture, the Band is let down under the Chin, to stay and strengthen its several Turns, and is terminated round the Head, in passing over the Fore-head.

If the Jaw be fractur'd on both sides, it wou'd be requisite to apply thereto a Bolster and Paste-board, perforated at the Chin, and of the Figure of the entire Jaw; the Bandage which we have even now describ'd, may be also prepar'd in making Rollers on both sides of the Jaw: Or else the double Chevestre may be made with a Band of five Ells long, and two Fingers broad, roll'd up with two Balls, that is to say, with the two Ends. The Application of this Band is begun under the Chin, from whence it is carry'd up over the Cheek, cross'd upon the top of the Head, and brought down behind the Head, where it is cross'd again; then it is let down under the Chin, cross'd there, and carry'd up over the Fracture; afterward the Band being pass'd three or four times over the same turns, in making Rollers upon the Jaws, is turn'd upon the Chin, and stay'd upon the Forehead round about the Head.

* * * * *

{276}

CHAP. III.

Of the Fracture of the Clavicle.

The Patient is to be set in a Chair, and his Arm is to be drawn backward, whilst an Assistant thrusts his Shoulder forward: In the mean time the Operator sets the Bones again in their place, by thrusting the Protuberances, and drawing out the sunk Bone.

Or else a Tennis-Ball may be taken, and put under the Patient's Arm-Pit, whose Elbow is then to be press'd against his Ribs, whilst the Surgeon reduceth the Fracture.

Otherwise, the Patient may be laid upon his Back, putting a Convex Body under both his Shoulders, as a Bowl, or large wooden Porrenger; and then the Shoulders may be prest, to raise up the two ends of the Bones, which the Surgeon must take care to reduce.

The Dressing and Bandage.

The Cavities which are above and below the Clavicle, are to be fill'd with Bolsters trimm'd with Paste-boards; another is to be also laid upon the Bone, which is almost of the same Figure with the Clavicle, and a large Bolster, to cover the three others: This Dressing is to be secur'd with the Bandage call'd the Capeline or Head-Bandage, provided the Fracture be in the middle of the Clavicle. A Band {277} being taken about six Ells long, and four fingers thick, roll'd with two Balls; it is apply'd in the middle to the Fracture; one of its Heads or Ends is let down upon the Breast, whilst the other is pass'd behind the Back, below the Arm-hole, opposite to the indispos'd Arm-hole and above the Breast, to be carry'd over the other end of the Band, which is rais'd up, to make a Roller or Bolster upon the Fracture: The other end is pass'd under the indispos'd Arm-pit, and upon the Band that made the Roller, which is elevated by making a third Roller upon the Clavicle: These Circumvolutions around about the Body are continu'd, as also these Rollers upon the Clavicle, till it be entirely cover'd. Some Circumvolutions are also made upon the upper part of the Arm, near its Head: The Space that lies between the Rollers and the Circumvolutions of the Arm, and which bears the Name of Geranium or Stork's-Bill, is likewise cover'd with some Circumvolutions, and the Band is stay'd by making Circumvolutions quite round about the Body.

If the Fracture were near the Head of the Humerus or Arm-Bone, a sort of Bandage might be prepar'd, which is call'd Spica, with a Band roll'd with one Ball five Ells long, and four fingers broad; one end of this Band is pass'd under the Arm-pit opposite to the indispos'd one behind the Back: The other end is convey'd under the indispos'd Arm-pit; the Figure of the Letters KY or X is made on the Shoulder; the Band is return'd below the other Shoulder behind; it is brought back again before, to form a second KY upon the {278} Fracture; three or four more KY's are wrought upon the Fracture; two Circumvolutions are made in the upper part of the Humerus, which constitute a Triangle call'd Geranium; this Triangle is cover'd with Rollers, and the Band is terminated round about the Breast.

* * * * *

CHAP. IV.

Of the Fracture of the Omoplata or Shoulder-Blade.

The Acromion is usually fractur'd, but it may be known that the middle of the Omoplata is broken by a Numness which is felt in the whole Arm: Whereupon the Surgeon, after having examin'd the place of the Fracture, thrusts back the Prominences of the Bones into their place; and if any Splints happen to prick the Part, he makes an Incision to take 'em out, or to cut off their Points.

The Dressing and Bandage.

A Bolster is laid upon the Omoplata, as also a large piece of Paste-board of the bigness and Figure of this Bone, and a sort of Bandage is prepar'd, known by the name of the Star, with a Band roll'd with one Head four Ells long, and as many Fingers broad. This Band is convey'd behind the Back, one of its ends lying under the Arm-hole, opposite to the indispos'd one; but the other is pass'd under the {279} Shoulder, and afterward above it, to make a KY in the middle of the Back; then passing under the other Arm-hole, it is brought up to the Shoulder, to be let down, and to form a second KY upon the middle of the Back: These Turns are continu'd in making Rollers, till the Omoplat?are all cover'd: Circumvolutions are also made round the upper part of the Humerus, as in the Spica; and the Bandage is finish'd by Circumvolutions round about the Breast.

* * * * *

CHAP. V.

Of the Fracture of the Ribs.

When a Rib is broken, one of the ends pusheth into the Breast, sometimes on the outside; and sometimes the Ends lie against each other. In order to reduce it, the Patient being laid upon the sound Rib, a Plaister of Mastick is apply'd to the Fracture; and it is drawn out violently; so that sometimes this Attraction brings back the Bone, which is advanc'd into the Breast; but the surest way is to make an Incision therein, to raise it up with the Finger.

If the Rib appear without, the Patient is to be set in a a Chair, and oblig'd to bend his Body on the side opposite to the Fracture, holding his Breath, with which he must puff strongly, without letting it forth, in order to dilate the Breast, whilst the Surgeon thrusts the Rib into its place.

{280}

The Dressing and Bandage.

A Bolster is to be apply'd to the Fracture, with two little Pieces of Pasteboard pass'd in form of a St. Andrew's Cross; and another Bolster upon the whole Dressing, on which is also laid a large square Paste-board cover'd with a Bolster. The Bandage is made with a Napkin folded into three Folds, which is put round the Breast, being sow'd and supported by the Scapulary; which is a Band six Fingers broad, perforated in the middle, to let in the Head. The two ends of the Scapulary are fasten'd before and behind to the Napkin.

* * * * *

CHAP. VI.

Of the Fracture of the Sternum or Breast-Bone.

To reduce this Fracture, the Patient is to be laid upon his Back, with a Convex Body underneath; both his Shoulders are to be press'd with some weight, to push 'em backward, and to raise up the Sternum, which is sunk down; or else an Incision may be made upon the Bone, to discover it; and then a Vectis is to be apply'd thereto very gently, in order to heave it up into its place.

{281}

The Dressing and Bandage.

A Bolster and Paste-board are to be laid upon the Sternum, almost of the same Figure with the Part; and the Bandage is to be prepar'd with a Napkin supported with a Scapulary. Or else the Bandage call'd Quadriga may be made with a Band roll'd with two Heads, five Ells long, and four Fingers broad: The Application of this Band is begun under the Arm-pit; the Figure of KY is form'd under the Shoulder; the Band is carry'd downward with the two Balls, once before, and the other behind; it is pass'd under the other Arm-hole; the Heads are cross'd upon the Shoulder, and it is brought down backward and forward, forming a KY before and behind. Afterward the Bank is roll'd about the Breast in making Rollers or Bolsters; these Rollers are continu'd till the Band be terminated; and it is stay'd by a Cirumvolution round the Breast.

* * * * *

CHAP. VII.

Of the Fracture of the Vertebra's.

The Apophyses of the Vertebra's are commonly broken, and their Bodies but seldom: It may be known that the Body of the Vertebra of the Neck and Back is fractur'd by the Palsie of the Arm, accompany'd with the loss of Feeling; by the suppression of Urine; {282} and by the Palsie of the Sphincter of the Anus; so that the Excrements cannot be any longer retain'd. If these Symptoms appear, it may well be conceiv'd that the Marrow is compress'd, and prickt with Points; for the removing of which, it is necessary to make an Incision upon the Body of the Vertebra in the fractur'd Place.

If the Apophyses Spinos?are only fractur'd, these Accidents will not happen, only some Pain will be felt: To reduce 'em, the Patient is to be laid upon his Belly, and the Surgeon must use his utmost endeavours to raise up the Bone again, and to set it in its Natural Situation.

The Dressing and Bandage.

If the Apophysis Spinosa were fractur'd, it wou'd be requisite to apply to each side of it a small long Bolster, which is to be cover'd with a Paste-board of the same Figure with the Bolster; another Bolster lying upon each Paste-board. The Bandage is to be made with a Napkin sustain'd by its Scapulary; or else the Quadriga may be prepar'd, according to the manner we have already describ'd in the Fracture of the Sternum.

* * * * *

{283}

CHAP. VIII.

Of the Fracture of the Os Sacrum.

It is reduc'd as the other Vertebra's; but its Dressing and Bandage are made with the T perforated at the Anus, or else with the H or double T. It is made with a Band two Fingers broad, and long enough to encompass the Body above the Hips; so that to the middle of this Band is fasten'd another Band of the same breadth, and of a sufficient length to pass over the Dressing of the Os Sacrum, as also between the Thighs, to be join'd in the fore-part to the first Cincture. The double T is made by fastening two Bands at a Finger's breadth distance one from another, to the Band which ought to be roll'd about the Body; and this sort of Bandage is to be supported with a Scapulary.

* * * * *

CHAP. IX.

Of the Fracture of the Coccyx or Rump-Bone.

This Bone is usually broken by falls, and sinks into the inside; so that to reduce it, the Fore-finger of one Hand is to be put into the Anus or Fundament as far as the {284} Fracture, to thrust it back again into its place, whilst the other Hand setleth it on the outside.

The Dressing and Bandage.

Are the same with those in the Fracture of the Os Sacrum; but the Patient must be oblig'd to lie on one side, and to sit in a perforated Chair, when he hath a mind to rise.

If the Os Innominatum be broken, the Spica is to be us'd after it hath been dress'd, of which Bandage we have given an Account in the Fracture of the Clavicle.

* * * * *

CHAP. X.

Of the Fracture of the Humerus or Arm-Bone.

To set this Bone, a strong Extension is to be made, if the two ends cross one another, to which purpose the Patient is to be plac'd on a little Stool or Seat, and supported by a Servant, two other Assistants being employ'd to draw, one at the upper-part, and the other at the lower, above the Elbow, and not beneath it. In the mean time the Operator reduceth the two Bones, by closing 'em on all sides with the Palms of his Hands, and afterward prepareth {285}

The Dressing and Bandage.

It is necessary at first to lay round the Fracture a Bolster steept in some proper Liquor, as Claret or Oxycratum; then three several Bands are to be taken, three or four Fingers broad, and an Ell and a half long: The first of these is to be laid upon the Fracture, round which are to be made three very streight Circumvolutions; then it is to be carry'd up with small Rollers to the top of the Arm, and stay'd round the Body. The second Band being apply'd to the Fracture, on the side opposite to the first, two Circumvolutions are to be made upon the Fracture; so that the same Band may be brought down along the whole length of the Arm, making divers Rollers, and at last stay'd below the Elbow, which, nevertheless, it must not cover. Afterward our Longitudinal Bolsters must be laid upon the Fracture round about the Arm, which are to be kept close with a third Band; it being of no great Importance whether the Application of this third Band be begun at the Top or at the Bottom; but it may be stay'd round the Body, or else beneath the Elbow. The Arm ought also to be encompass'd with two thick pieces of Paste-board made round at the ends, and of the length of the Arm; but they must not cross one another. These Paste-boards are to be fasten'd with three Ribbands, and the Arm is to be put into a Scarf made with a large Napkin, which is to be first apply'd in the middle under the Arm-pit, the Arm resting upon it, so that {286} the four ends may be rais'd up, and fasten'd to the opposite Shoulder; but the Hand must lie higher than the Elbow.

* * * * *

CHAP. XI.

Of the Fracture of the Bone of the Elbow.

If both the Bones of the Elbow be broken, a stronger Extension is to be made than if only one of 'em were so hurt; to which purpose a Servant is to be appointed to grasp the Arm above the Elbow with both his Hands, and another to hold it above the Wrist, whilst the Surgeon sets the Bones with the Palms of both his Hands, till no unevenness be any longer felt in the Part.

The Dressing and Bandage

Are the same with those in the Fracture of the Arm; but the Bands which are carry'd upward are to be stay'd above the Elbow. If the Patient be desirous to keep his Bed, it is requisite that his Arm be laid upon a Pillow, the Elbow lying somewhat higher than the Hand.

* * * * *

{287}

CHAP. XII.

Of the Fracture of the Carpus or Wrist-Bone.

If the Bones of the Carpus, or those of the Metacarpium be fractur'd, a Servant must hold the Arm above the Wrist, and another the Fingers; whilst the Operator sets the Bones in their place, so as no unevenness may appear in the Part.

The Dressing and Bandage.

Of the Fracture of the Wrist are to be prepar'd with a Band roll'd with one Head, being six Ells Long, and two Fingers broad; so that three Circumvolutions are to be made upon the Wrist; the Band is to be pass'd over the Hand, between the Thumb and the Fore-finger, making the Figure of KY upon the Thumb. Then after having made divers Rollers upon the Carpus, a Bolster is to be apply'd, with a little Piece of Paste-board of the same Shape with the Wrist; several Rollers are to be form'd on the top of the Elbow, to stay the Band above it; and the Arm is to be put into a Scarf.

* * * * *

{288}

CHAP. XIII.

Of the Fracture of the Bone of the Metacarpium.

Two Servants are to hold the Hand, after the same manner as in the setting of the Carpus or Wrist-Bone, whilst the Surgeon reduceth the broken Bone by fixing it in its Natural Situation.

The Dressing and Bandage

Are made with a Band roll'd up with one Head, five Ells long, and two Fingers broad: This Band being fasten'd to the Wrist, with a Circumvolution, is to be laid on the Metacarpium, between the Thumb and the Fore-finger, and the Figure of KY is to be made upon the Hand: Then the forming of Rollers and KY's is to be continu'd till the Metacarpium be cover'd; a Bolster and Paste-board are to be laid upon the same Metacarpium; as also one in the Hand, of the Shape of the Part: The inside of the Hand is to be trimm'd; and the whole Contexture is to be cover'd as before, with Rollers; which are continu'd till above the Elbow, where the Band is stay'd.

* * * * *

{289}

CHAP. XIV.

Of the Fracture of the Fingers.

A Light Extension is to be made in the Fingers to reduce 'em, and a small Dressing is to be prepar'd for every Finger, almost like that of the Arm. The Fingers are to be somewhat bent, and the inside of the Hand is to be trimm'd with a Bolster, to retain 'em in this Situation. The Bolster is also to be stay'd with a Band, and the Arm to be put into a Scarf.

* * * * *

CHAP. XV.

Of the Fracture of the Thigh.

If the Thigh-Bone be broken near its Head, the Fracture is very difficult to be discover'd; but if the Bone pass one over another, it may be soon known, because the hurt leg will be shorter than the other. Therefore a very great Extension is to be made; and if the Hands are not sufficient for that purpose, recourse may be had to Straps and Engines. In the mean time the Operator is to lay his Thumbs upon the fractur'd Bone, to thrust it back into its place, and afterward to apply {290}

The Dressing and Bandage.

The Cavity of the Thigh is to be fill'd with a thick Bolster, of the length of its bending; and three Bands four Fingers broad are to be provided, the first being three Ells long, and the second four, as well as the third: Then three Circumvolutions are to be made upon the Fracture with the first Band, carrying it up with small Rollers, and it is to be stay'd round the Body. The second Band is to make two Circumvolutions upon the Fracture, and is to be brought down with small Rollers, which are terminated above the Knee; or else they may be continu'd all along the Leg; it is also to be pass'd under the Foot, and to be drawn up again upon the Leg: Then a Bolster is to be apply'd to the lower part of the Thigh, being thicker at bottom than at top, to render the Thigh everywhere even; and four Longitudinal Bolsters are to be added, on which are laid Splints of the same length and breadth, which are to be wrapt up with a single Bolster. The third Band is to be roll'd upon these Splints, beginning at the bottom, and ascending with Rollers. Then two large Paste-boards are to be us'd, which may embrace the whole Dressing, without crossing one another, being fasten'd with three Ribbands. Afterward a Pair of Pumps is to be put under the Foot, and the Heel to be supported with a small Roll, the Thigh and Leg being let into the Scarves, the inner of which is to extend to the Groin, and the {291} outermost is to be somewhat longer: Two little Cushions are also to be laid on each side below the Knee, and two others below the Ankles, to fill up the Cavities. These Cushions or large Bolsters are to lie between the Scarves; and a thick Bolster is to be laid upon the Leg all along its length, as also on upon the Thigh. The Scarves are to be bound with three Ribbands for the Legs, and as many for the Thighs; the Knots being ty'd without, and on the side.

* * * * *

CHAP. XVI.

Of the Fracture of the Knee-Pan.

The Knee-Pan is cleft or broken in divers pieces in its length, and cross-wise: If it be broken cross-wise or obliquely, the two Pieces fly out one from another; and on this occasion a strong Extension is to be made; whilst the Surgeon at the same time thrusts back again the upper-part of the Knee-Pan into its place.

If the Knee-Pan be fractur'd in its length, no Extension can be made, because the pieces of the Bones remain in their place.

The Dressing and Bandage.

If the Knee-Pan be broken cross-wise, a Band is to be provided three Ells long, and two Fingers Broad, which may be roll'd with {292} one or two Heads. The Application is to be begun above the Knee-Pan; the Figure of KY is to be made in the Ham, and a Circumvolution under the Knee; then the Band is to be continually carry'd up and down, till the Knee-Pan be entirely cover'd.

If the Knee-Pan be fractur'd in its length, that is to say, from the top to the bottom, the Uniting-Band must be us'd, being two or three Ells long, and two Fingers broad, perforated in the middle. It is to be at first apply'd under the Knee, and one of the Balls is to be pass'd thro' the Hole; it must also be well clos'd, and divers Circumvolutions are to be made upon the Knee-Pan, so as it may be altogether cover'd.

* * * * *

CHAP. XVII.

Of the Fracture of the Leg.

If the Tibia be only broken, it pushes into the Inside; but if both Bones be fractur'd they are sometimes separated on both sides, or else they pass one upon another; and in this case the Leg is shorter than it ought to be. If the Perone be broken, it pushes to the outside.

If one Bone be only fractur'd, so strong an Extension is not requisite as when they are both shatter'd, and it is to be drawn only on one side; whereas the drawing ought to be equal on both sides when both Bones are concern'd. {293} Thus whilst the Assistants are employ'd in drawing, the Surgeon performs the Operation, by laying the ends of the Bones exactly against one another; and they are known to be reduc'd when the great Toe remains in its Natural Situation.

The Dressing and Bandage.

A simple Bolster dipt in a convenient Liquor is at first apply'd, and three Bands three Fingers broad are prepar'd, the first being two Ells long, the second three, and the third three and a half. Three very streight Circumvolutions are to be made upon the Fracture; the Band is also to be carry'd up with Rollers, and stay'd above the Knee. The Application of the second Band is to be begun upon the Fracture with two Circumvolutions; it is to be brought down with Rollers, to pass under the Foot, afterward carry'd up again, and stay'd where it is terminated. The Leg is to be fill'd with a Bolster thicker at the bottom than at the top; and then are to be laid on the four longitudinal Bolsters, two Fingers broad, and as long as the Leg; to which are to be apply'd the Splints of a plyable and thin Wood: These are wrapt up with a simple Bolster, and strengthen'd with the third Band, which is apply'd indifferently either at the top or bottom, opposite to the former; so that it is carry'd up or else down in making Rollers, and stay'd at its end. The whole Contexture is to be encompass'd with large Paste-boards made round at the Ends, which are not to cross one another, {294} but must be streighter at the bottom than at the top, and are to be ty'd with three Ribbands or pieces of Tape, beginning at the middle; so that the Knots be ty'd on the outside. Afterward the Leg is to be put into the Scarves, and the Heel is to be supported with a Linnen-Roll, to which are fasten'd two Ribbands that are ty'd upon the Scarves: These Rolls are made with a small piece of Cloth, which is doubl'd, and roll'd up with the ends, in which is contain'd some Straw, and a little Stick in the middle, to consolidate 'em. The Foot is supported with a Paste-board or Wooden Sole, trimm'd with a Bolster, or small Quilt sow'd over it. Divers Strings are also fasten'd to the middle of the sides of the Sole or Pump, which are cross'd to be joyn'd to the Scarves; and another is fixt at the end of the Sole, which is ty'd to a Ribband that binds the middle of the Scarf. These Scarves are likewise fasten'd with three Ribbands, beginning with that in the middle, the Knots being without, and trimm'd with four Bolsters, that is to say, two on each side, to fill up the Cavities that are below the Knee, and above the Ankle. Lastly, the Leg is to be plac'd somewhat high, and a Cradle to be laid upon it, to keep off the Bed-Cloaths, the Scarves passing over the Knee and Foot.

The Dressing of Complicated Fractures

Of the Arms, Legs, and Thighs is prepar'd with a Bandage having Eighteen Heads or Ends, in order to make which, a Linnen-Cloth is to {295} be taken of the length of the Part, and broad enough to cause it to be cross'd thereby: It is to be folded into three doubles, and cut in three places on each side, leaving the middle plain; so that eighteen Heads or small Bands are form'd, every one of which will be four fingers broad, the upper Heads being a little shorter than the lower. This Band of eighteen Heads is to be laid upon the

Scarves, and a Bolster is to be apply'd to it four Fingers broad, as long as the Scarves. The Leg is laid upon this Bolster, and it hinders the corrupt Matter from falling on the Bandage.

When the Wound hath been dress'd, the fracture is to be incontinently surrounded with one of the Heads, which ought to cross one another: Then after the Leg hath been bound with the first Heads, two Longitudinal Bolsters are to be apply'd to the side of it; and the other Heads are to be rais'd up, with all the rest of the Dressing, which hath been describ'd in the simple Fracture.

* * * * *

CHAP. XVIII.

Of the Fracture of the Bone of the Foot.

The Reduction of the Bone of the Foot is perform'd after the same manner as that of the Hand. {296}

The Dressing and Bandage

Are made with a Band roll'd with two Heads, being three Ells long, and two Fingers broad: The Application of it is begun with a Circumvolution above the Ankles; it is pass'd on the Foot, and in like manner makes a Circumvolution round it: Afterward the same Band is cross'd over the Metatarsus, upon which are made some Folds in form of a Rhombus or Diamond; as also on the Toes, and it is stay'd above the Ankle-Bone; or else it is carry'd up along the Leg, to be stay'd above the Knee. This Bandage serves for all Fractures of the Bones of the Foot, and is call'd the Sandal.

* * * * *

{297}

A

TREATISE

OF THE

OPERATIONS

Which are perform'd in

LUXATIONS.

* * * * *

CHAP. I.

Of the Luxation of the Nose.

The Bones of the Nose may be separated from that of the Fore-head by a Fall, or some violent Blow; and the Surgeon in order to set 'em, at first lays his Thumb upon the Root of the Nose, and then he introduceth a little Stick trimm'd with Cotton, into the Nostrils, and by the means thereof thrusts back the Bones into their place. {298}

The Dressing and Bandage

Are the same with those that have been already describ'd in the Fracture of the Bones of the Nose.

* * * * *

CHAP. II.

Of the Luxation of the lower-Jaw.

The Jaw may be luxated either on both sides, or only on one. When the Dislocation happens on both sides, it hangs over the Sternum or Breast-Bone, and the Spittle runs abundantly out of the Mouth: To reduce it, the Patient must sit down, and his Head is to be supported by a Servant; then the Operator or Surgeon having wrapt up his two Thumbs, puts 'em into the Mouth upon the Molar Teeth, his other Fingers lying under the Jaw, which is to be drawn down by raising it up, having before set two small Wooden Wedges upon the two Molar Teeth on both sides of the Jaw, lest the Surgeon's Fingers shou'd be hurt, as the Bone is returning to its place.

If the Luxation be forward, a Band or Strap is to be put under the Chin, an Assistant having his Knees upon the Patient's Shoulders, where he is to draw the Strap upward, to facilitate the Extension; which the Surgeon makes with his Hands, at the same time thrusting the Bone back again into its place. {299}

When the Jaw is luxated only on one side, the Chin stands a-cross, and the dislocated side is squash'd down, a small Cavity being perceiv'd in it, and a Rising on the other side; so that the Mouth cannot be shut close, but remains somewhat open, the lower Teeth appear farther out than the upper; and the Canine or Dog-Teeth lie under the Incisive. This Luxation is reduc'd by giving a blow with the Hand upon the luxated Bone, which is sufficient to cause it to re-enter its Natural Place.

The Dressing and Bandage

Are altogether the same with those us'd in the Fracture of the Bones of the lower Jaw.

* * * * *

CHAP. III.

Of the Luxation of the Clavicle.

The Clavicle is oftner loosen'd from the Acromion than from the Sternum; when it hath left the former the Arm cannot be lifted up; the Acromion makes a Prominence, and the Clavicle descends downward, a Cavity appearing in its place. To reduce this Luxation, the Patient is to be laid upon some Convex Body put between his Shoulders; both which are to be press'd backward, to raise up the Clavicle: Afterward he is to be set in a Chair, that his Arm may be drawn backward, whilst the {300} Surgeon is employ'd in pressing the Clavicle and Acromion, to join 'em together.

The Dressing and Bandage

Are the same with those that we have already shewn, in treating of the Fracture of the Clavicle.

* * * * *

CHAP. IV.

Of the Luxation of the Vertebra's.

In the Luxation of the Vertebra's of the Neck, the Head stands to one side, and the Face is swell'd and livid, with a difficulty of Respiration.

To reduce this Dislocation, the Patient is to be set upon a low Seat, an Assistant leaning on his Shoulders, to keep his Body steady, whilst the Surgeon or Operator draws his Head upward, and turns it from one side to another: Then if the Accidents or Symptoms cease, the Cure is perform'd; so that Fomentations may be apply'd to the Part; and the Patient being laid in his Bed, must take care to avoid moving his Head.

When the Vertebra's of the Back or Loins are luxated on the inside, a sinking of the Bone is soon perceiv'd; whereupon the Patient being laid on his Belly, the Extension is to be made with Napkins pass'd under the Arm-Pits, and upon the Os Ileum, whilst the Surgeon with {301} a strong Extension makes some Efforts on the Spine, endeavouring to draw back the Vertebra. If that be not sufficient, an Incision is to be made upon the Apophysis Spinosa of the Vertebra; so that after having laid open this Process of the Bone, it may be taken out with a Pair of Forceps. Then the Wound is to be dress'd with Pledgets, a Plaister, and a Napkin, which must not be bound too close, for fear of pushing back the Spine.

When the Vertebra is luxated on the outside, a Prominence appears; so that to reduce this Dislocation, the Extension is to be made as before, the Patient lying in like manner upon his Belly; but in order to push back the Vertebra, two little Sticks trimm'd with Linnen-Cloth are to be prepar'd, and laid along the two sides of the Spine of the Vertebra; yet these Sticks ought to be thick enough to remain more elevated than the Apophysis Spinosa; and a large wooden Roller is to be often roll'd upon 'em, which by its turning backward and forward, may thrust the Vertebra's inward; so that when all the Vertebra's are of an equal height, the Reduction is finish'd. If the Vertebra's are luxated on the side, the same Extensions are to be made, and the Prominence is to be push'd, to re-establish the Vertebra in its place.

The Dressing and Bandage.

The Dressing is prepar'd by laying two thin Plates of Lead on each side of the Spinous Process of the Vertebra, to maintain it in its Place, and a long Bolster over 'em. The {302} proper Bandage is the Quadriga, which hath been before describ'd, in treating of the Fractures of the Breast-Bone.

* * * * *

CHAP. V.

Of the Luxation of the Coccyx or Rump-Bone.

If the Coccyx be sunk on the inside, it is to be rais'd with the Fore-finger of the Right-hand put into the Anus; and if the Luxation be on the outside, it may be gently thrust back again. An Account of its proper Dressing and Bandage hath been already given in the Fracture of the Coccyx.

* * * * *

CHAP. VI.

Of the Bunch.

The Bunch is nothing else but an exterior Luxation of the Vertebra's, and for the Cure thereof, it wou'd be requisite to keep Emollients for a long time upon the Vertebra's, to loosen the Ligaments, and to wear Iron-Bodice; which in compressing the Vertebra's by little and little, might perhaps drive 'em back into their Natural Place.

* * * * *

{303}

CHAP. VII.

Of the Luxation of the Ribs.

The Ribs are luxated either on the outside, or on the inside: If they be dislocated on the inside, a Cavity is perceiv'd near the Vertebra's, the Patient drawing his Breath with Pain, and not being able to bend his Body.

When the Luxation is on the outside, and happens in the upper Ribs, the Patient's Hands are to be hoisted upon the top of a Door, to raise up the Ribs, whilst the Surgeon presseth the Prominence of the Rib to restore it to its place.

When the lower Ribs are luxated, the Patient must be oblig'd to stoop, laying his Hands upon his Knees, and the Prominence of the Bone is to be thrust back.

If a Rib be luxated on the inside, an Incision is to be made to draw it out with the Fingers.

The Dressing and Bandage

Are the same with those that are us'd in the Fracture of the Ribs.

* * * * *

{304}

CHAP. VIII.

Of the Sinking of the Xiphoides, or Sword-like Cartilage.

To raise up the Xiphoid Cartilage, it must be fomented before for some time with Oil of Turpentine, or other Fomentations, made with Aromaticks; then the Patient is to be laid upon his Back, with a Convex Body underneath, and the Shoulders, and Sides of the Breast are to be press'd, to lift up the Cartilage. When this Operation is not sufficient, dry Cupping-Glasses are usually apply'd, till the Part be elevated, and a strengthening Plaister is afterward laid upon it.

* * * * *

CHAP. IX.

Of the Luxation of the Humerus, or Arm-Bone.

The Head of the Humerus generally falls under the Arm-Pit, so that the luxated Arm becomes longer than the other, the Acromion appears pointed on the outside; the Elbow starts from the Ribs, and cannot be mov'd without great Pain. To reduce this Bone, the {305} Patient is to be set upon a low Seat, or else on the Ground, whilst some Person supports his Body with a Napkin: In the mean time the Surgeon is to lay hold on the upper-part of the Humerus, a Servant kneeling behind him, who is to hold the Patient's Arm above the Elbow, which is to pass between the Surgeon's Legs, and is to be drawn down by the Assistant as much as is possible, whilst the Surgeon in like manner draws the Arm, to remove the Head of the Bone out of the place where it was stopt; insomuch that the Bone sometimes makes a Noise in re-entring its Cavity.

Or else the Patient's Arm may be laid upon the Shoulder of a taller Man than himself, who is strongly to draw the luxated Arm upon the Fore-part of his Breast; during which time, the Operator is to push the Head of the Humerus, to cause it to re-enter its Cavity.

Otherwise the Patient may lie on the Ground, a Tennis-Ball being put under his Arm-Pit, which a Servant is to draw strongly with a Handkerchief pass'd under the Shoulder, whilst another Assistant stands behind the Patient, to thrust down the Shoulder with his Foot; at the same time the Surgeon sitting between the Patient's Legs, is to push strongly with his Heel the Ball that lies under the Arm-hole.

Or else, a thick Battoon or Leaver may be laid on the Shoulders of two Men, after a Tennis-Ball hath been nail'd on the middle of it; otherwise a Bunch may be made therein, and cover'd with Linnen-Cloth; two Wooden Pins being also fixt on each side of the Ball: {306} Then the Patient's Arm-Pit is to be set between those two Pins, and upon the Ball, where he is to remain hanging, whilst his Arm is pull'd down by main force. The same thing may be done by laying the Patient's Arm-Pit upon a Door, or else upon the Round of a Ladder.

The Dressing and Bandage

A little Ball of Linnen is to be laid under the Arm-Pit, and underneath a Bolster with four Heads, which are cross'd upon the Shoulder; as also a Bolster under the sound Arm-Hole, that it may not be gall'd by the Bandage Spica, the Nature of which we have shewn in treating of the Fracture of the Clavicle.

* * * * *

CHAP. X.

Of the Luxation of the Elbow.

When the Elbow is luxated on the inside, the Arm flies out, and the Hand is turn'd outward; but in the Luxation on the outside, the Arm is shortned: If the Luxation be Lateral, a Prominence appears in the Dislocated, and a Cavity in the opposite Part.

To reduce the Internal Luxation, the Humerus and Cubitus are drawn, and at the same time the Surgeon bends the Elbow, by carrying {307} the Hand toward the Shoulder; or else a Tennis-Ball may be laid in the Fold of the Elbow, and the Arm drawn toward the Shoulder.

For the External Luxation, the Extension is to be made, whilst the Surgeon thrusts back the Elbow into its place: Or else a round Stick may be taken, and trimm'd with Linnen-Cloth, with which the Bone is to be push'd back into its place during the Extension. This Stick may be also us'd in the reducing of the Internal Luxation.

For the Lateral Luxations, the Extension may be made in like manner; the Surgeon at the same time thrusting back the Bone into its Natural Situation.

The Bandage

Is made with a Band five Ells long, and two Fingers broad, roll'd with one Ball: The Application of it is begun with a Circumvolution at the lower part of the Humerus, it is pass'd over the Fold of the Arm; a Circumvolution is also form'd in the upper-part of the Elbow, and the Figure of KY in its Fold. Afterward the Rollers are continu'd upon the Elbow, and the KY's in the inside of the Arm, till the Elbow be entirely cover'd: The Band is likewise carry'd up to the top of the Arm with Rollers, and stay'd round about the Body. The Patient must be oblig'd to keep his Bed, or else his Arm may be put in a Scarf, after the same manner as in the Fracture of the Arm.

* * * * *

{308}

CHAP. XI.

Of the Luxation of the Wrist.

If the Luxation be Internal, the Hand is turn'd back to the outside, so that for the Reduction thereof, it wou'd be requisite to cause the back of the Hand to be laid upon a Table, and the Extension to be made by drawing the Elbow and Hand, whilst the Surgeon takes care to press the Prominence.

If the Luxation be External, the Hand is bended on the inside; so that to reduce it, the inside of the Hand is to be laid upon a Table, and the Surgeon is to press it after the Extension.

If the Luxation be on the sides, the Hand is turn'd to one side; so that the Extension must be made, and the Hand turn'd on the side opposite to the Luxation. But the Fingers are usually drawn one after another, to the end that the Tendons may be set again in their Place.

The eight Bones of the Carpus may be in like manner dislocated both on the inside and without; and to set 'em right, the Hand is to be laid upon a Table, and the Extension to be made, so as to press the Protuberances on the inside, if the Luxation be internal, and on the outside if it be external. {309}

The Bandage

Is prepar'd with a Band six Ells long, and two Fingers broad; so that three Circumvolutions may be made upon the Luxation; as also divers Rollers in passing thro' the inside of the Hand between the Thumb and the Forefinger, and in forming the Figure of KY upon the Thumb, after having made many Rollers upon the Wrist. Two Pieces of Paste-board are also to be laid on the sides of the Wrist, which are bound with the same Band in making Rollers; and the Hand is to be trimm'd with a Linnen-Ball, to keep the Fingers in their mean Situation. Then the Band is to be pass'd above, to strengthen it, and carry'd up with Rollers along the whole length of the Elbow, to be stay'd below the same Elbow.

* * * * *

CHAP. XII.

Of the Luxation of the Fingers.

If the Fingers be luxated, it is necessary to make an Extension to reduce 'em, and afterward to use the following

Bandage.

If the Luxation be in the first Articulation or Joint, the Bandage Spicais to be apply'd, being made of a Band roll'd with one Head, an {310} Ell long, and an Inch broad: It is begun with Circumvolutions round about the Wrist, and brought over the Luxation in passing between the Fingers. These Circumvolutions are also continu'd to form a Spica upon the Luxation; and the Band is stay'd at the Wrist.

If all the first Phalanges were dislocated, it wou'd be requisite to make as many upon every Phalanx, and with the same Band: This sort of Bandage is call'd the Demi-Gantlet.

* * * * *

CHAP. XIII.

Of the Luxation of the Thigh.

The Luxation which most commonly happens in this Part, is the Internal; so that a Protuberance appears on the Hole of the Os Pubis; the indispos'd Leg is longer than the other, and the Knee and Foot turn outward; neither can the Thigh be any longer bended, nor drawn near the other.

If the Luxation be External, the Leg becomes shorter than the other, the Knee and Foot turning inward, and the Heel to the outside.

When the Luxation is on the fore-part, a Tumour ariseth in the Groin, so that the Patient cannot draw this Thigh toward the other, nor bend the Leg; his Body resting only upon the Heel.

{311}

If the Luxation be Posterior, a Tumour is felt in the Buttocks with great Pain, and the Legg is shorter than it ought to be: There also appears a sinking in the Groin, the Leg is lifted off from the Ground, and the hurt Person is apt to fall backward.

To reduce the Internal Luxation, the Patient is to be laid with his Back upon a Table, to which is fixt a thick Wooden Pin, about a Foot long, which is to be set between his Thighs, to detain his Body when his Legs are drawn down; then a Strap is to be pass'd above the joynt of the Thigh, to draw the Ischion upward; and the Thigh is to be drawn down with another Strap fasten'd above the Knee: In the mean while the Surgeon thrusts the Thigh upward, to cause it to re-enter its Cavity, the Straps being somewhat loosen'd in the time of the Reduction to facilitate the Operation.

To reduce the External Luxation, the Patient is to be laid upon his Belly; and the drawing to be perform'd after the same manner as we have even now shewn, whilst the Thigh is thrust from the outside inward, to cause the bone to re-enter its Cavity.

In reducing the Anterior Luxation, the hurt Person is to be laid upon the side opposite to the Luxation, and Extensions are to be made, by drawing both upward and down-ward, as before: Then the Head of the Bone is to be forc'd, by the means of a Ball thrust strongly with the Knee, in drawing the luxated leg toward the other. {312}

The Posterior Luxation is thus reduc'd; The Patient being laid upon his Belly, the double Extension is to be made, and his Knee drawn outward, to set the Bone in its place. After the Operation hath been perform'd, a Bolster is to be apply'd, steept in Spirituous Medicaments; and the Bandage call'd Spica, of which we have given an Account in treating of the Luxation of the Shoulder.

* * * * *

CHAP. XIV.

Of the Luxation of the Knee.

When the Tibia is luxated behind, its Prominences are in the Cavity of the Ham, and the Leg flies off, or is bended. If the same Tibia be dislocated on the side, a kind of Tumour appears in the luxated side, and a Sinking in the opposite. But if the Condylus of the Tibia remains in the inside, the Leg turns outward; and if it be in the outside, it turns inward.

The Posterior Luxation is reduc'd by obliging the Patient to lie upon his Belly, whilst the Surgeon during the Extensions bends the Leg, in drawing the Heel toward the top of the Thigh.

If the Tibia be luxated on the side, the usual Extensions are to be made, and the Bone is to be push'd with the Knee. {313}

If the Luxation were in the fore-part, it wou'd be requisite to lay the Patient upon his Back, to make the Extensions, by drawing the Thigh and Leg; and to press the protuberant Parts.

The Bandage

Is prepar'd with a Band three Ells long, and two Fingers broad, roll'd with two Balls: A Circumvolution being at first made above the Knee, the Figure KY is form'd underneath, and a Circumvolution above it; then the Band is carry'd up again over the Knee, in making Rollers and KY's underneath, till the Knee be entirely cover'd.

* * * * *

CHAP. XV.

Of the Luxation of the Patella or Knee-Pan.

The Knee-Pan is luxated by starting upward; and to reduce it, the Patient's Leg is to be held streight, whilst it is thrust back into its place with the Hands. Then he must be oblig'd to keep his Bed; and the same Bandage is to be apply'd with that which hath been describ'd for the Luxation of the Knee.

If the Perone or Fibula be remov'd from the Tibia, the sides of the Foot are to be press'd, to draw it back again; and it may be kept close {314} with the Bandage which is appropriated to the Fractures of the Tarsus.

The Astragalus may be also luxated in the fore-part; so that the Operator ought to thrust it back into its place, and to make use of the Bandage which we have prepar'd for the Fracture of the Foot.

The Calcaneum sometimes flies off from the Astragalus both in the inside and without; and the Bones of the Tarsus, Metatarsus, and Toes are likewise apt to be luxated. But a little Circumspection is only requisite to reduce all these Dislocations.

* * * * *

{315}

A

TREATISE

OF

Medicinal Compositions

Necessary for a

SURGEON.

* * * * *

CHAP. I.

Of Balsams.

* * * * *

The Balsam of Arc 鎢 s.

Take two Pounds of the Suet of a He-Goat, Venice Turpentine and Gum Elemi, a Pound and a half of each; and of Hogs-Lard one Pound. After the Gum Elemi, being cut into small Pieces, hath been melted over a very gentle Fire, add to it the Turpentine, Goats-Suet, and {316} Swines-Grease; and when all these Ingredients are well dissolv'd, strain the Liquor thro' a new Linnen-Cloth, to separate the Scum and Dregs from it; then let the whole Mass cool, and the Balsam is made.

This Balsam serves to incarnate and consolidate all sorts of Wounds and Ulcers: It is likewise us'd in Fractures and Dislocations of the Bones; as also to cure the Contusions and Wounds of the Nerves.

The Balsam of Spain.

Take pure Wheat, the Roots of Valerian and Carduus Benedictus, of each one Ounce, and beat 'em well in a Mortar with a Pint of White-Wine; strain the whole Composition into an Earthen Vessel Leaded, having a narrow Mouth; stop up the Vessel, and set it upon hot Embers during twenty four Hours: Then add six Ounces, of St. John's Wort; set the whole Mass in Balneo Mari? till the Wine be consum'd and let it be strain'd and squeez'd. Afterward add two Ounces of Frankincense well pulveriz'd, with eight Ounces of Venice Turpentine, mixing 'em together over a gentle Fire, and the Balsam will be made.

This is the Balsam which was always us'd by Hieronymus Fabritius ab Aguapendente, a noted Italian Surgeon, and is excellent for all kinds of Wounds, even for the Nervous, which (as it is avouch'd by some Persons) may be cur'd by it within the space of twenty four Hours. But the Wound must be at first wash'd with good White-Wine cold, and afterward anointed {317} with this Balsam well heated. If the Wound be deep, it may be syringed with the same Balsam very hot, and the sides of it anointed when drawn together. Then a Bolster steep'd in the Balsam is to be apply'd to the Part, and upon that another Bolster soakt in the Lees of Wine; as also over this last another drie Bolster.

The Green Balsam.

Take Linseed-Oil and that of Olives, of each one Pint; one Ounce of Oil of Bays; two Ounces of Venice Turpentine, half an Ounce of the destill'd Oil of Juniper-Berries, three Drams of Verdegrease, two Drams of Sucotrin Aloes, two Drams and a half of White Vitriol, and one of the Oil of Cloves.

Having made choice of the best Olive and Linseed-Oil well purify'd and mingl'd together in a Skillet or Pan over a very gentle Fire, let the Turpentine and Oil of Bays be incorporated in it; then having taken off the Pan from the Fire, and left the Liquor to be well cool'd, let it be intermixt by little and little with the Verdegrease, the White Vitriol, and the Sucotrin Aloes beaten to fine Powder: Afterward the destill'd Oils of Cloves and Juniper-Berries being added, and the whole Composition well mingl'd together, the Balsam will be entirely compounded according to Art.

This is the Balsam that hath been so much talkt of at Paris, and which many Quack-Salvers, pretending to the Art of Physick and Surgery, keep as a great Secret. Indeed it is very good for all sorts of Wounds, whether they {318} be made by the Sword, or other Iron Weapons, or by Gun-shot. But it wou'd be requisite at first to wash the Wound with warm Wine, then to anoint it with this Balsam very hot, and to apply Bolsters that have been steept in it, as also a large Bolster over the other, dipt in some Styptick Liquor. This Balsam mundifies, incarnates, and cicatrizes Wounds; being likewise good against the Bitings of venomous Beasts, and fistulous and malignant Ulcers.

Samaritan Balsam.

Take an equal quantity of common Oil and good Wine; boil 'em together in a glaz'd Earthen Vessel, till the Wine be wholly consum'd, and the Balsam will be made. I have produc'd this Balsam in particular, by reason of its simplicity, and in regard that it may be readily prepar'd at all times. It serves to mundifie and consolidate simple Wounds more especially those that are recent.

* * * * *

{319}

CHAP. II.

Of Ointments.

* * * * *

Unguentum.

Take of the Roots of Marsh-Mallows, six Ounces, the Seeds of Line, and Fenugreek, and Squills, of each four Ounces; of yellow Wax one Pound; Colophony and Rosin, of each one Pound; Venice Turpentine, Galbanum, and Gum Heder?pulveriz'd, two Ounces of each. The Marsh-Mallow-Roots being newly gather'd, are to be well wash'd and slic'd, as well as the Squills. After they have been put into a Copper-Pan or Skillet, tinn'd over on the inside, together with the Seeds of Line and Fenugreek, and a Gallon of fair Water pour'd upon 'em, the whole Mass is to be macerated during twenty four Hours, over a very gentle Fire, stirring the Ingredients from time to time with a Wooden Spatula: Thus they are to be boil'd slowly, often reiterating the stirring, till the Mucilages are sufficiently thicken'd; then, after having well squeez'd and strain'd 'em thro' a strong and very close Cloth, and mingl'd 'em with the prepar'd Oil, they are to be boil'd together again over a very gentle Fire, till the Superfluous Moisture of the Mucilages be wholly {320} consum'd: Afterward having strain'd the Oil again, the yellow Wax, Colophony, and Rosin cut into small pieces, are to be melted in it; and if any Dregs appear at the bottom of the Pan, when the whole Mass is dissolv'd, it is to be strain'd a-new, or at least the pure Liquor must be separated from the gross or impure by Inclination, whilst it is as yet very hot: The Ointment is to be stirr'd about with a Wooden Pestle; and when it begins to grow thick, you may add the Turpentine, the Galbanum purify'd and thicken'd, and the Gum Heder?beaten to fine Powder, all which Ingredients were before incorporated together. Then the Ointment is to be continually stirr'd, till it be altogether grown cold.

This Ointment serves to moisten, mollifie, and heat gently; it also allayes the Pains of the Side, and softens Tumours, particularly the Parotides. It may be us'd either alone, or with other Ointments or Oils.

The mundificative Ointment of Smallage.

Take three handfuls of Smallage-Leaves; with Ground-Ivy, great Wormwood, great Centory, Germander, Sage, St. John's-Wort, Plantain, Milfoil or Yarrow, Perewinkle, the greater Comfrey, the lesser Comfrey, Betony, Honey-suckle, Fluellin, Vervein, Knot-Grass, Adders-Tongue, and Burnet, of every one of these Plants two handfuls; a Gallon of common Oil, white Pitch, Mutton-Suet, yellow Wax, and Turpentine, of each two Pounds. {321}

Bruise all these Herbs in a Marble-Mortar; let the Wax, white Pitch, and Mutton-Suet cut into pieces, as also the Turpentine be melted in the Oil, in a Copper-Pan lin'd with Tin, over a moderate Fire; put the bruis'd Herbs in it, and cause the whole Mass to simmer together very slowly, stirring it about from time to time with a Wooden Spatula. As soon as it shall be perceiv'd that the Oil of the Herbs is almost quite consum'd, the whole Composition is to be strain'd, and strongly squeez'd. Then after having let the Ointment cool, to draw off all the Dregs and Moisture, it is to be dissolv'd over a very gentle Fire; and after having left it a little while to cool again and thicken, you may add thereto Myrrh, Aloes, FlorenceOrris, and round Birth-Wort pulveriz'd very fine. When all these Ingredients are by this means well incorporated, the Ointment will be brought to perfection.

This Ointment is of singular Use to cleanse Ulcers; as also to mundifie, cicatrize, and consolidate all sorts of Wounds.

The black or suppurative Ointment.

Take a Quart of common Oil, white and yellow Wax, Mutton-Suet that lies near the Kidneys, pure Rosin, Ship-Pitch, Venice Turpentine, of each half a Pound; and of Mastick beaten to fine Powder, two Ounces; let all that is capable of being dissolv'd, be liquify'd in the Oil; and add the Powder of Mastick to make an Ointment. {322}

This Ointment searches and opens all sorts of Impostumes, as well as Carbuncles, and Pestilential and Venereal Bubo's. The use of the same Ointment is also to be continu'd after the opening of the Abcesses, till their perfect Cure be compleated.

Unguentum Rosatum.

Take Bore's-Grease well purify'd, and often wash'd, and Red Roses newly pickt, of each four Pounds, with the like quantity of White Roses.

The thin Membrane or Skin which lies upon the Bores-Grease, being taken away, it is to be cut into small pieces, well wash'd in fair Water, and melted in a glaz'd Earthen-Pot over a very gentle Fire; the first Grease that is dissolv'd is to be strain'd thro' a Cloth, well wash'd, and mixt with the same quantity of thick Rose-Buds well bruis'd. Then the whole Mass is to be put into a glaz'd Earthen-Pot with a narrow Mouth; the Pot is to be well stopt, and set during six Hours in Water, which is between luke-warm and boiling hot. Afterward it is to be boil'd an Hour, strain'd and strongly squeez'd. In the mean while four Pounds of White Roses newly blown are to be taken, well bruis'd, and mingl'd with the former Composition, the Pot being cover'd, which is likewise set for the space of six Hours in Water, between luke-warm and boiling hot: Then the Liquor is to be strain'd and strongly squeez'd. Lastly, after the Ointment hath been cool'd, and separated from its F鎡 es or Dregs, it may be kept for use. {323}

If it be desir'd to give a Rose-Colour to this Ointment, it wou'd be requisite a quarter of an Hour before it be strain'd the last time, to throw into it two or three Ounces of Orcanet, which is to be stirr'd into the Ointment. If it be thought fit to retain the White Colour, and to produce the smell of Roses, it may be done with Damask-Roses without Orcanet. If you are desirous to give it the Consistence of a Liniment, you may add Oil of sweet Almonds to the quantity of a sixth part of its weight.

This Ointment is a very good Remedy against all manner of external Inflammations, particularly against Phlegmons, Erysipelas's, and Tetters; as also against the Head-ach and H 鎚 orrhoids or Piles.

Unguentum Album, aut de Cerussa.

Take three Pints of Oil of Roses, nine Ounces of white Wax, one Pound of Venice Ceruse or white Lead, and a Dram and a half of Camphire.

The Ceruse being pulveriz'd by rubbing the pieces upon the Cloath of a Hair-Sieve turn'd upside-down; the Powder is to be receiv'd on a Sheet of Paper laid underneath, and to be often wash'd with Water in a great Earthen-Pan, stirring it about with a Wooden Spatula, and pouring off the Water by Inclination as soon as the Powder is sunk to the Bottom. When the Water of these Washings grows insipid, the last Lotion is to be made with Rose-Water, leaving it for the space of five or six Hours, which being expir'd, it is to be pour'd off by Inclination, and {324} the Ceruse must be dry'd in the Shade, cover'd with Paper. Then the broken Wax and prepar'd Oil is to put into a glaz'd Earthen-Pot, and the Pot into the boiling Bath. As soon as the Wax is melted, the Pot may be taken out of the Bath, and the dissolv'd Liquor stirr'd with a Wooden Pestle till it begins to grow thick. Afterward the pulveriz'd Ceruse is to be infus'd, and the Ointment stirr'd about till it be almost cold. If you shall think fit to add Camphire, let it be dissolv'd in a little Oil, and incorporated with the Ointment when it is cold. The Whites of Eggs may be also well mixt with the Ointment, by stirring it about, to make an exact union of the several Ingredients.

This Ointment is good for Burns, Erysipelas's, the Itch, and many Distempers of the Skin; it allayes the Itchings and intemperature of Ulcers; it dissipates the Chafings and Redness that happen in the Bodies of Infants; It is of great efficacy in the healing of Contusions, and it serves to consolidate and cool light Wounds.

Unguentum.

Take eleven Ounces of Verdegrease, fourteen Ounces of strong Vinegar, and twenty eight Ounces of good Honey.

Let the Verdegrease be put into a Copper-Pan or Skillet over a very gentle Fire; then bruise it with a Wooden Pestle; work it well in the Vinegar, and strain the whole thro' a Hair-Sieve. If a little Verdegrease remains on the Sieve, it is to be put again into the {325} Skillet bruis'd and beaten small therein, as before, with a Portion of the same Vinegar, straining it thro' the Sieve, till the unprofitable drossy parts of the Copper be only left. Afterward this Liquor is to be boil'd over a gentle Fire, with the Honey, stirring it about from time to time till it hath acquir'd the Consistence of a softish Ointment, and a very red Colour.

This Ointment consumes putrify'd Flesh, and the Superfluities of Ulcers and Wounds.

Unguentum Basilicon, or Royal Ointment.

Take yellow Wax, Mutton-Suet, Rosin, Ship-Pitch, and Venice Turpentine, one Pound of each; with five Pints of common Oil.

Cut the Suet, Rosin, and black Pitch into small Pieces, and let 'em be melted together, with the Oil, in a Copper-Pan over a very moderate Fire; then after having strain'd the Liquor thro' a thick Cloth, let it be incorporated with the Turpentine, and the Ointment will be made.

It promotes Suppuration, and cicatrizes Wounds when the purulent Matter is drawn forth. It is often laid alone upon the Bolsters, and sometimes mixt with the Yolks of Eggs, Turpentine, and other Ointments, or with Oils and Plaisters. {326}

A cooling Cerate.

Take a Pint of Oil of Roses, and three Ounces of white Wax.

Let the whole Composition be put into a glaz'd Earthen-Pot, and the Pot set in Balneo Mari? till the Wax be well dissolv'd in the Oil: Then take the Vessel out of the Bath, and stir the Ointment with a Wooden Pestle till it be cool'd; add two Ounces of Water, and stir it about with the Pestle till it be imbib'd by the Cerate; let as much more Water be infus'd, and again the same quantity, till the Cerate becomes very white, and hath been well soakt with fresh

Water. Afterward all the Water is to be pour'd off by Inclination, and separated as much as is possible from the Cerate, which may then be kept for use; but some Surgeons cause an Ounce of Vinegar to be mingl'd with it.

This Cerate is usually laid outwardly upon all Parts that stand in need of cooling, and asswages the Pains of the Hemorrhoids or Piles. It is also good for Chaps, sore Nipples, and other ill Accidents that happen in the Breast; and is us'd for Burns either alone, or mixt with other Ointments. Whensoever it is necessary to apply Desiccatives and Astringents to any Part, this Cerate may be mingl'd with Unguentum de Cerussa. {327}

An Ointment for Burns.

Take a Pound of Bores-Grease, two Pints of White-Wine, the Leaves of the greater Sage, Ground- and Wall-Ivy, Sweet Marjoram, or the Greater House-Leek, of each two handfuls.

Let the whole Mass be boil'd over a gentle Fire, and having afterward strain'd and squeez'd it, let the Ointment so made be kept for use.

* * * * *

CHAP. III.

Of Plaisters.

* * * * *

The Plaister of Diapalma.

Take three Pounds of prepar'd Litharge of Gold, three Pints of common Oil, two Pounds of Hogs-Lard, a Quart of the Decoction of Palm-Tree or Oak-Tops; four Ounces of Vitriol calcin'd till it become red, and steept in the said Decoction. Having bruis'd or cut very small two handfuls of Palm-Tree or Oak-Tops, let 'em be boil'd slowly in three Quarts of Water till about half be consum'd; and after the whole Mass hath been well squeez'd, the strain'd Decoction is to be preserv'd. In the mean time the Litharge is to be {328} pounded in a great Brass Mortar, and diluted with two or three Quarts of clear Water; but it will be requisite readily to pour out into another Vessel the muddy Water which is impregnated with the more subtil part of the Litharge, whilst the thicker remains at the bottom of the Mortar; whereupon this part of the Litharge will sink to the bottom of the Water, and the Litharge remaining in the Mortar is to be pounded again. Then having diluted it in the Water of the first Lotion, or in some other fresh Water, the muddy Liquor is to be pour'd by Inclination upon the subtil Litharge that remain'd in the bottom of the Vessel: Afterward you may continue to pound the Litharge, to bruise it in the Water, to pour it off by Inclination, and to let the Powder settle, till there be left only at the bottom a certain impure part of the Litharge, capable of being pulveriz'd, and rais'd amidst the Water. As soon as the Lotions are well settl'd, and care hath been taken to separate by Inclination the Water which swims over the Powder of Litharge; this Powder is to be dry'd, and having weigh'd out the appointed Quantity, it is to be put as yet cold into a Copper-Pan lin'd with Tin, and stirr'd about to mingle it with the Oil, Lard, and Decoction of Palm-Tree-Tops. When these Ingredients have been well incorporated together, a good Charcoal Fire must be kindl'd in a Furnace, over which they are to be boil'd, stirring 'em continually with a great Wooden Spatula, and constantly maintaining an equal Degree of Heat during the whole time of their boiling. At last you may add {329} the rubify'd Vitriol dissolv'd in a Portion of the Liquor that hath been reserv'd, if you wou'd have the Plaister tinctur'd with a red Colour; or else white Vitriol melted in the same Decoction, if it shall be thought fit to retain the Whiteness of the Plaister, which may be form'd into Rolls, and wrapt up with Paper.

This Plaister is us'd for the cure of Wounds, Ulcers, Tumours, Burns, Contusions, Fractures, and Chilblains, and is also laid upon the Cauteries. If you mingle with it the third or fourth part of its weight of some convenient Oil, it will attain to the Consistence of a Cerate; and this is that which is call'd Dissolved Diapalma or Cerate of Diapalma.

The Plaister of simple Diachylum.

Take of Marsh-Mallow-Roots peel'd, three Drams; the Seeds of Line and Fenugreek, of each four Ounces; three Quarts of Spring-Water; two Quarts of common Oil, and two Pounds of Litharge of Gold.

Let the Mucilages of Marsh-Mallow-Roots, and of the Seeds of Line and

Fenugreek be taken, as hath been shewn in the making of Unguentum, and let the Litharge be prepar'd after the same manner as for the Plaister of Diapalma. Having at first well mixt the Oil with the Litharge in a large Copper-Vessel or Pan, Tinn'd on the inside, being wide at the top, and tapering like a Cone toward the bottom, as also having afterward added and well incorporated the Mucilages, a moderate {330} Charcoal Fire is to be kindl'd in a Furnace, upon which the Vessel is to be set, and the whole Mass is to be stirr'd about incessantly with a Wooden Spatula; and as fast as is possible. A gentle Fire is to be maintain'd, and the Boiling and Agitation to be continu'd, till it be perceiv'd that the Plaister begins to sink in the Pan; then the Heat of the Fire must be diminish'd one half at the least; and it will be requisite only to cause an Evaporation by little and little, of the Superfluous Moisture that might remain in the plaister, which being consum'd, it will be sufficiently boil'd, having attain'd to its due Consistence and Whiteness.

This Plaister softens and dissolves hard Swellings, and even the Scirrhous Tumours of the Liver and Bowels; such are the Scrophulous or King's-Evil Tumours, the old remains of Abcesses, &c.

The Plaister of Andreas Crucius.

Take two Ounces of Rosin; four Ounces of Gum Elemi, Venice Turpentine and Oil of Bays, of each two Ounces.

After having beat in pieces the Rosin and Gum Elemi, they are to be melted together over a very gentle Fire, and then may be added the Turpentine and Oil of Bays. When the whole Mass hath been by this means well incorporated, it must be strain'd thro' a Cloth, to separate it from the Dregs. The Plaister being afterward cool'd, is to be made up in Rolls, and kept for use.

{331}

This Plaister is proper for Wounds of the Breast: It also mundifies and consolidates all sorts of Wounds and Ulcers, dissipates Contusions, strengthens the Parts in Fractures and Dislocations, and causeth the Serous Humours to pass away by Transpiration.

Emplastrum Divinum.

Take of Litharge of Gold prepar'd, one Pound and an half; three Pints of common Oil; one Quart of Spring-Water; six Ounces of prepar'd Load-Stone; Gum Ammoniack, Galbanum, Opoponax, and Bdellium, of each three Ounces; Myrrh, Olibanum, Mastick, Verdegrease, and round Birth-Wort, of every one of these an Ounce and an half; eight Ounces of Yellow Wax, and four Ounces of Turpentine.

Let the Gum Ammoniack, Galbanum, Bdellium, and Opopanax be dissolv'd in Vinegar, in a little Earthen Pipkin; strain 'em thro' a course Cloth, and let 'em be thicken'd by Evaporation, according to the Method before observ'd in other Plaisters: Then prepare the Load-Stone upon a Porphyry or Marble-Stone, and take care to bruise separately, the Olibanum, the Mastick, the Myrrh, the round Birth-Wort, and the Verdegrease, which is to be kept to be added at last. In the mean while, having incorporated cold the Oil with the Litharge, and mingl'd the Water with 'em, they are to be boil'd together over a very good Fire, stirring 'em incessantly, till the whole Composition hath aquir'd the Consistence of a somewhat solid {332} Plaister, in which is to be dissolv'd the yellow Wax cut into small pieces. Afterward having taken off the Pan from the Fire, and left the Ingredients to be half cool'd, intermix the Gums, which have been already thicken'd and incorporated with the Turpentine; then the Load-Stone mingl'd with the Birth-Wort, Myrrh, Mastick, and Olibanum; and last of all the Verdegrease. Thus when all these Ingredients are well stirr'd and mixt together, the Plaister will be entirely compounded; so that it may be made up into Rolls, and preserv'd to be us'd upon necessary Occasions.

This Plaister is efficacious in curing of all kinds of Wounds, Ulcers, Tumours, and Contusions; for it mollifies, digestes, and brings to Suppuration such Matter as ought to be carry'd off this way. It also mundifies, cicatrizes, and entirely consolidates Wounds, &c.

* * * * *

CHAP. IV.

Of Cataplasms or Pultisses.

Cataplasms are usually prepar'd to asswage Pain; as also to dissolve and dissipate recent Tumours, and are made thus:

Take four Ounces and a half of white Bread, one Pint of new Milk, three Yolks of Eggs, one Ounce of Oil of Roses, one Dram of Saffron, and two Drams of the Extract of Opium.

{333}

The Crum is to be taken out of the inside of a white Loaf newly drawn out of the Oven, and to be boil'd with the Milk in a Skillet over a little Fire, stirring it from time to time with a Spatula, till it be reduc'd to a thick Pap. After having taken the Vessel off from the Fire, the three Yolks of Eggs beaten are to be put into it, and the Dram of Saffron pulveriz'd; to these Ingredients may be added two Drams of the Extract of Opium somewhat liquid, if the Pain be great.

Here is another Cataplasm proper to mollifie and to bring to Suppuration when it is necessary.

Take White-Lilly-Roots, and Marsh-Mallow-Roots, of each four Ounces; the Leaves of common Mallows, Marsh-Mallows, Groundsel, Violet-Plants, Brank-Ursin, of every one of these Herbs one handful; the Meal of Line, Fenugreek, and Oil of Lillies, of each three Ounces.

The Roots when wash'd and slic'd, are to be boil'd in Water, and the Leaves being added some time after, the Boiling is to be continu'd till the whole Mass becomes perfectly tender and soft; at which time having strain'd the Decoction, beat the remaining gross Substance in a Stone-Mortar, with a Wooden Pestle, and pass the Pulp thro' a Hair-Sieve turn'd upside-down: Then let the Decoction and Pulp so strain'd be put into a Skillet, and having intermixt the Meal of Line, Fenugreek, {334} and Oil of Lillies; let 'em be boil'd together over a gentle Fire, stirring about the Ingredients from time to time, till they be all sufficiently thicken'd. These two Cataplasms may serve as a Model for the making of many others.

* * * * *

CHAP. V.

Of Oils.

Oils are made either by Infusion or Expression.

Simple Oil of Roses made by Infusion.

Take two Pounds of Roses newly gather'd, and bruis'd in a Mortar; half a Pint of the Juice of Roses, and five Pints of common Oil: Let the whole Composition be put into a Earthen-Vessel, Leaded and well stopt, and then let it be expos'd to the Sun during forty Days. Afterward let it be boil'd in Balneo Mari? and having strain'd and squeez'd the Roses, let the Oil be kept for use.

Compound Oil of Roses made by Infusion.

Take a Pound of Red Roses newly gather'd, and pound 'em in a Mortar; as also four Ounces of the Juice of Red Roses, and two Quarts of common Oil. Let the whole Composition be put into an Earthen-Vessel Leaded, the Mouth {335} of which is narrow, and well stopt; and then having expos'd it to the Sun during four Days, let it be set in Balneo Mari?for an Hour, and then strain'd and squeez'd. Afterward let this Liquor be put into the same Vessel, adding to it the Juice of Roses, and Roses themselves, in the same quantity as before: Let the Vessel be stopt; let the Maceration, Boiling, Straining, and Expression be made in like manner as before; and let the same Operation be once more re-iterated: Then let your Oil be depurated, and preserv'd for use.

These Oils qualifie and disperse Defluctions of Humours, suppress Inflammations, mitigate the Head-ach and Deliriums, and provoke to sleep. They must be warm'd before the Parts are anointed with 'em, and they may be given inwardly against the Bloody-flux and Worms, the Dose being from half an Ounce to a whole Ounce. The Parts are also anointed with 'em in Fractures and Dislocations of the Bones, and Oxyrodins are made of 'em with an equal quantity of Vinegar of Roses.

Oil of Sweet Almonds made by Expression.

Take new Almonds that are fat and very dry, without their Shells, and having shaken 'em in a somewhat thick Sieve, to cause the Dust to fall off; let 'em be put into hot Water till their Skins become tender, so that they may be separated by squeezing 'em with the Fingers: Afterward having taken off the Skin, they must be wip'd with a white Linnen-Cloth, and spread upon it to be dry'd: Then they are {336} to be put into a Stone-Mortar, and pounded with a Wooden-Pestle, till the Paste grows very thin, and begins to give Oil: This Paste is to be put into a little Linnen-Bag, new and strong, the Mouth of which hath been well ty'd; and the Bag is to be plac'd between two Platines of Tin, or of Wood lin'd on the inside with a Leaf of Tin, squeezing the whole Mass gently at first; but afterward very strongly, and leaving it for a long while in the Press, that the Oil may have time to run out.

This Oil mitigates the Nephritick Colicks, remedies the Retention of Urine, facilitates Child-birth, allayes the After-Pains in Women after their delivery, and the Gripes in young Infants: It is taken inwardly fasting from half an Ounce to two Ounces; and it is us'd in Liniments to asswage and mollifie. The Oils of common Wall-Nuts and Small-Nuts, may be also prepar'd after the same manner as that of Sweet-Almonds.

The Oil of Bayes.

Take as much as you please of Laurel or Bay-Berries, well cleans'd, perfectly ripe, and soundly bruis'd; let 'em be put into a Kettle, and boil'd with a sufficient quantity of Water during half an Hour; then strain and squeeze 'em strongly; let the Liquor cool, and scum off the Fat that swims upon the Water: Afterward pound the remaining Substance in a Mortar, and cause it to be boil'd again for half an Hour, with some of the first Water which was left, adding a little fresh; then strain and squeez it, {337} as before, and take off the Oil that swims on the Top. But the first Oil is better than the second, and therefore ought to be kept separately. The Oils of Berries of Mastick, Myrtle, and other oleaginous Plants, may be extracted after the same manner.

The Oil of Bayes mollifies, attenuates, and is opening and discussive: It is very good against the Palsie, and the Shiverings or cold Fits of a feaver or Ague in anointing the Back; as also against Scabs, Tetters, &c.

The Oil of Eggs by Expression.

Take newly laid Eggs, and let 'em be harden'd in Water; then separate the Yolks, and put 'em into a Frying-pan over a gentle Coal-fire, stirring 'em about from time to time, and at last without discontinuing, till they grow reddish, and begin to yield their Oil: Then they are to be sprinkl'd with Spirit of Wine, and pour'd very hot into a little Linnen-Bag, which is to be ty'd, and set in a Press between two heated Platines; so that the Oil may be squeez'd out as readily as is possible.

This Oil mitigates the Pains of the Ears and Hemorrhoids, cures Scabs and Ring-Worms or Tetters; as also Chaps and Clefts in the Breast, Hands, Feet, and Fundament; and is made use of in Burns, &c.

* * * * *

{338}

CHAP. VI.

Of Collyrium's.

Collyrium's are Medicines prepar'd for the Diseases of the Eyes: The following is that of Lanfrancus.

Take a Pint of White-Wine, three Pints of Plantain-Water, three Pounds of Roses, two Drams of Orpiment, one Dram of Verdegrease; Myrrh and Aloes, of each two Scruples.

The Orpiment, Verdegrease, Myrrh, and Aloes are to be beaten to a fine Powder before they are intermixt with the Liquors. This Collyrium is not only good for the Eyes, but is also of use to make Injections into the Privy-Parts of Men and Women; but before the Injections are made, it ought to be sweeten'd with three or four times the quantity in weight of Rose, Plantain, or Morel-Water.

A dry Collyrium.

Take two Drams of Sugar-candy; prepar'd Tutty, Lizard's-Dung, of each one

Dram; White Vitriol, Sucotrin Aloes, and Sal Saturni, of each half a Dram.

Let the whole Composition be reduc'd to a very fine Powder, and mixt together: Two or three Grains of this Powder may be blown at {339} once into the Eye with a small Quill, Pipe of Straw, or Reed, as long as it is necessary; and the same Powder may also be steept in Ophthalmick Waters, to make a liquid Collyrium.

A Blue Collyrium.

Take a Pint of Water in which unslackt Lime has been quench'd, and a Dram of Sal Ammoniack pulveriz'd; mingle these Ingredients together in a Brass-Bason, and let 'em be infus'd during a whole Night; then filtrate the Liquor and keep it for use.

This Collyrium is one of the best Medicines that can be prepar'd for all manner of Diseases of the Eyes.

* * * * *

CHAP. VII.

Of Powders.

* * * * *

A Powder against Madness or Frenzy.

Take the Leaves of Rue, Vervein, the lesser Sage, Plantain, Polypody, common Wormwood, Mint, Mother-Wort, Balm, Betony, St. John's-Wort, and the lesser Centory; of every one an equal quantity.

These Plants must be gather'd in the Month of June, during the clear and serene Weather, {340} and ty'd up in Nose-gays, or little Bundles; which are to be wrap'd up in Paper, and hung in the Air to be dry'd in the Shade. Afterward they are to be pounded in a great Brass-Mortar, and the Powder is to be sifted thro' a Silk-Sieve.

The Dose of this Powder is from two to three Drams, mingl'd with half a Dram of the Powder of Vipers, in half a Glass of good White-Wine every Morning fasting, for fifty one Days successively. It has an admirable effect, provided the wounded Person be not bit in the Head nor Face, and that the Wound has not been wash'd with Water.

* * * * *

CHAP. VIII.

Styptick-Water.

Take Colcothar or Red Vitriol that remains in the Retort after the Spirit has been drawn off, Burnt Allom, and Sugar-candy, of each thirty Grains; the Urine of a Young Person, and Rose-Water, of each half an Ounce; and two Ounces of Plantain-Water: Let the whole Mixture be stirr'd about for a long time, and then put into a Vial. But the Liquor must be pour'd off by Inclination when there shall be occasion to take any for use. {341}

If a Bolster steept in this Water be laid upon an open Artery, and held close with the Hand, it will soon stop the Blood; a small Tent may be also soakt in it, and put up into the Nose for the same purpose. If it be taken inwardly, it stops the spitting of Blood, and the Dysentery or Bloody-Flux; as also the Hemorrhoidal and Menstruous Fluxes; the Dose being from half a Dram to two Drams, in Knot-Grass-Water.

* * * * *

FINIS.

www.ingramcontent.com/pod-product-compliance
Lightning Source LLC
Chambersburg PA
CBHW070852180526
45168CB00005B/1791